HOW MUCH DO YOU REALLY KNOW ABOUT NUTRITION AND YOUR CHILD'S HEALTH?

TRUE OR FALSE:
- Raisins cause cavities quicker than soda
- Children who eat six small meals a day are less likely to be overweight
- 13-year olds have the worst diet of any age group
- Children *don't* have to eat vegetables to be healthy
- Young athletes need extra protein
- Children who skip breakfast don't perform as well on tests

"Information-packed, highly accessible guide to enjoyable meals and healthy children."
—*ALA Booklist*

"Public libraries will want this book."
—*Library Journal*

"A thorough, informative, and reassuring guide for parents . . . sound nutrition advice that's easy to follow."
—Judith Nolte, Editor
American Baby Magazine

"I've never known anyone who gave more supportive or realistic nutrition advice to parents."
—Ruth Pleva, Executive Director
Pleva Center for Childbirth
Education and Family Counseling

Books by Annette B. Natow and Jo-Ann Heslin

Megadoses
No-Nonsense Nutrition for Kids

Published by POCKET BOOKS

NO-NONSENSE NUTRITION FOR KIDS

Annette Natow & Jo-Ann Heslin

PUBLISHED BY POCKET BOOKS NEW YORK

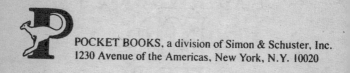

POCKET BOOKS, a division of Simon & Schuster, Inc.
1230 Avenue of the Americas, New York, N.Y. 10020

Published by arrangement with McGraw-Hill, Inc.
Library of Congress Catalog Card Number: 84-7149

ISBN: 0-671-60779-0

First Pocket Books printing January, 1986

10 9 8 7 6 5 4 3 2 1

To all our children,
who brought us joy and knowledge.

Feeding must be a matter of principle not of impulse, and the reward will be partly in the present—much more in the future.

MARY SWARTZ ROSE,
FEEDING THE FAMILY, 1919

ACKNOWLEDGMENTS

We would like to thank the following people for all their assistance:

Carol Roche, Ph.D., Eugenia and Emmanouel Lambrinos, Lucretia Steele, Stanley Salvatore, Irene Rosenberg, M.D., and Laura Lefkowitz for typing the manuscript; and our families, Harry, Allen, Laura, Steven, Marty, Joseph, Kristen, and Karen, for their assistance, support, and encouragement.

Contents

**Part II—Nutritional Needs in
Special Situations**

Appendices

Preface

Getting children to eat healthy and nutritious foods can be a difficult and frustrating job. We are convinced, however, that good nutrition translated into choosing good food and establishing good eating habits is the most important contribution you can make to insure the health of your child. This book will help you to make the best possible food choices and to cope with the changes in your growing child's body and activities that affect what he or she eats. You may be confused by some of the things you read and hear about food. Our aim is to acquaint you with basic nutrient needs so that you can then decide, intelligently, what foods are best for your child.

We strongly believe that there are many ways to be well nourished. Therefore, we offer numerous options, never rules. We have always believed in moderation and flexibility. Our children were never tempted by a sprout and avocado sandwich on wheat berry bread served with carrot juice! Why should yours be any different? Good nutrition can be provided in the average American home without using special foods, excessive vitamins, or protein supplements. We'll show you how.

The answers we give to questions are loaded with ideas for action. We won't spend endless paragraphs explaining the physical and mental ramifications of a skipped breakfast; instead we will give you ideas to get your child to eat in the morning.

The book is divided into three parts. Part I explains the nutritional needs of the growing child, ages 1 to 13. Part II will focus on problems common to children of these ages— feeding during illness, dental health, weight control, feeding the junior athlete, and allergies. Part III offers some "kid-tested" recipes.

Many of the topics, such as snacking, will be covered in each chapter under every age group. This is where the index will prove very helpful. It will guide you to *all* the questions that discuss snacking. Many times a question answered for an older or younger child will give you ideas you can use.

The appendices were designed to provide a wealth of information to serve as an additional resource.

We hope to help you handle this most important time in your child's life.

To your child's health!

Part I

Nutrition and the Growing Child

One

Feeding a Toddler (Ages 1 to 3)

"Children learn methodically.
First they touch, then they look,
*then they taste . . . tasting is important to learning. . . ."**

About the time your baby reaches his first birthday, he may also be taking his first steps. This is an important milestone for you and for baby. He is becoming more independent and your infant is now a toddler. This sense of independence often spills over into mealtimes. Just when you thought you were becoming an expert in the care and feeding of your baby, he's changed. You don't know what to expect next. Your toddler is a bundle of contradictions . . .

He has teeth . . . but won't chew!

He explores . . . but won't try new foods!

* From a poster by Growing Child, P.O. Box 620, Lafayette, Indiana 47902.

He's interested in food . . . but would rather play with it than eat it!

He spoons up food expertly . . . but can't get it in his mouth!

He drinks from a cup . . . but spills or tips the cup daily!

He eats two servings of beans today . . . but won't touch them tomorrow!

Besides his changeable behavior with food, your toddler is changing in other ways. His growth has slowed down. In his first year he grew 10 inches and tripled his weight while in the next *two* years he will grow only about 6 inches and gain 9 pounds. That's why he no longer is the eager eater he was. A reduced appetite is usual in children after their first birthday. Even though they are active, they need less food because their growth is slower. And because his appetite is smaller, you must be sure that he gets all the nutrients he needs in the small amounts of food he *will* eat. That means that you must be careful how you choose and prepare the foods.

At the same time that you are providing good food choices you should also be encouraging good eating habits that will form the foundation for a lifetime of good health. This may sound like a tall order, but you can do it. The following often-asked questions and their answers will help you deal with the problems you are likely to have. After you read them, you will be able to plan mealtimes and snacktimes that both you and your toddler will enjoy.

At the end of the chapter, we have questions for *you*. Your answers will help you to judge for yourself how well you are doing.

DAILY NEEDS

Q *Is there a guide I can use so I will know what foods my toddler should eat each day?*

The Daily Food Guide for the Toddler, page 6, can help you. A good way to be sure that you are serving nutritious meals and snacks to your toddler is to choose one food from each of the four food groups for each meal and one food from each of two food groups for snacks. Here's an example:

Breakfast
  4 oz. orange juice
  1 scrambled egg
  ½ slice whole wheat toast
  ½ cup of milk

Lunch
  1 open-faced grilled cheese sandwich
  ½ banana
  ½ cup milk

Dinner
  1 little hamburger
  ¼ cup mashed potato
  2 tablespoons carrots
    graham cracker
  ½ cup milk

Snacks
      Afternoon   *Bedtime*
  ¼ cup apple juice   ½ cup milk
  1 bread stick   oatmeal cookie

These are just suggestions—try them.

Daily Food Guide for the Toddler

A toddler needs daily:

Milk
    2 cups
    1 serving = ½ cup

Use whole milk, evaporated milk (reconstituted with water), skim milk, nonfat dry milk, buttermilk, cheese, yogurt.

Meat, Fish, Poultry, and Protein-Rich Foods
    2–3 servings
    1 serving = 1 ounce*

Egg, cheese, dried peas or beans, tofu, peanut, and other nut butters may be substituted for a serving of meat, fish, or poultry.

Vegetables and Fruits
    4 or more servings
    1 serving of vegetable = 2–3 tablespoons
    1 serving of fruit   = ½ fresh fruit or
                             ¼ cup cooked or canned fruit

1 serving vitamin C–rich source (orange, grapefruit, melon, strawberries, broccoli, tomatoes, coleslaw).
1 serving of a vitamin A–rich food, dark green or deep yellow-orange in color (spinach, sweet potato, carrot, apricot, mango).
2 or more servings of other fruits and vegetables (including potatoes).

Bread, Cereal, Rice, Pasta
    3–4 servings
    1 serving = ½ slice bread
              = ¼ cup cooked cereal, pasta, or rice
              = ½ ounce or ⅓–½ cup dry cereal

Use only whole grain and enriched products.

* See page 7 for portion sizes of 1 ounce of protein.

Q *How big is the actual serving size for 1 ounce of protein?*

An ounce of a protein food gives your child about 7 grams of protein. A toddler needs approximately 23 grams of protein each day. Each of the following equals a 1-ounce serving and 7 grams of protein:

    1 hamburger (2 inches diameter × ½ inch thick)
    1 meatball (1 inch diameter)
    1 slice meat, chicken, turkey (2 inches × 2 inches × ¼ inch thick)
    1 cube of stew meat (1 inch square)
    1 cube cheese (1 inch square)
    1 slice cheese
    1 slice luncheon meat
    ½ frankfurter*
    ¼ cup cottage cheese
    1 medium egg
    2 tablespoons peanut butter
    ½ cup dried peas or beans
    3 ounces of tofu (soybean curd)
    3 tablespoons peanuts*

* Not recommended for children under the age of 3.

Q *I have heard that fiber is important for adults. Is it good for my toddler too?*

Fiber is an important part of a balanced diet, but it really isn't necessary for you to make a special effort to be sure your child gets enough of it. If he usually eats whole grain breads and cereals like whole wheat bread, rye bread, corn bread, oatmeal bread, oatmeal cereal, shredded wheat, or puffed wheat along with fruit and vegetables, your toddler probably has enough bulk. Breads with high fiber content like sprouted wheat or with sunflower seeds added may be irritating to the small child's digestive tract. In most cases it is neither necessary nor desirable to add additional fiber in the form of unprocessed bran to your young child's foods. The use of fiber in the diet of the constipated child will be discussed in Chapter 5.

BREAST- AND BOTTLE-FEEDING

Q *My mother insists that nursing my 16-month-old is wrong. Is that so?*

Absolutely not! Do not let your mother's opinion persuade you to stop nursing. Breast-feeding declined in popularity in the last 20 years but lately it has become popular again. As more women nurse, more women will continue to nurse longer and breast-feeding a toddler will not be unusual.

The decision to *start* nursing and the decision to *stop* is yours. Many women nurse a few months and stop, others have successfully nursed their children to age three. Extended nursing is common in many cultures. As long as you and your toddler remain a "contented couple" there is no reason to stop breast-feeding.

Q *Can you suggest how I should wean my toddler?*

Weaning means "to coax or move gradually from one type of feeding to another." It should be accomplished slowly. Abrupt weaning can be painful for you since milk production does not stop simply because you've decided not to nurse any longer. Milk production took time to initiate; it will also take time to terminate. We would recommend a "weaning month."

Start by dropping one breast-feeding a day. A midday feeding is most convenient since the breasts are most full in the morning and the evening feeding provides a great deal of comfort to the child. Substitute a cup of whole milk for this feeding. After four or five days drop another breast-feeding, substituting with whole milk once again. When the breast-feedings number one a day, begin nursing at this feeding only enough to remove the sensation of fullness. After a week of one feeding a day, start to skip days between feedings unless your breasts are uncomfortably full. Milk production has dropped off markedly by this time and you will find yourself forgetting to breast-feed. At this point weaning is complete.

Q *I'm pregnant. Can I continue to breast-feed my toddler?*

Yes. Pregnancy and breast-feeding can go hand in hand as long as you eat well, get sufficient rest, and your weight gain is normal. A nursing toddler really gets more security and psychological benefits from nursing than he gets nourishment.

Tandem nursing, new infant and toddler, is also possible, though demanding on you. If you should consider doing this, contact your local LaLeche League for further information. Check under LaLeche League in the white pages of your phone directory or contact their national office: LaLeche League International, Inc., 9616 Minneapolis Ave., Franklin Park, Illinois 60131.

Q *My 18-month-old still wants a bottle. How can I discontinue the bottle?*

For many children the need to suck and the sucking reflex persists well into the second year of life. Every child is an individual with his own unique timetable for development. An independent baby may discard his bottle early, yet another child may cling to his bottle as he would a favorite toy.

Respect your toddler's individuality. If he gains satisfaction from the bottle and is reluctant to let it go, let him keep it. If you feel uncomfortable with a toddler "bottle-in-tow," set limits on the use of the bottle. A toddler will accept his milk in a cup at meals if he knows his morning juice and prebedtime milk will appear in a bottle—a compromise between what you find acceptable and your toddler's needs.

A word of caution: To prevent dental caries, *never* put your toddler to sleep with a bottle, unless it is filled only with plain water. (For more information on dental health, see Chapter 6.)

MEALTIME MANNERS

Q *How can I make mealtime with my toddler more pleasant?*

There are lots of things that you can do so that both you and your toddler will enjoy mealtimes. Some of these are just plain common sense. It's important to recognize that your child needs fairly regular meals offered at close enough intervals so that he isn't too hungry to enjoy eating. Most toddlers do well with four or five meals and snacks daily. On the other hand, food offered too soon after the child has eaten is likely to be refused.

Your child should eat in a cheerful place, one that is clean, bright, airy, and fresh smelling, the same sort of place where you would enjoy eating. Most people enjoy company when they eat. So does your toddler. Avoid a lot of activity at mealtime that might be distracting, as it could be more interesting than the food. A child who has been playing actively all morning needs 10 or 15 minutes of quiet time to help him relax before eating.

The foods served should be chosen so that they have interesting shapes, different textures, and make a pleasing color combination. Try to include some finger foods. It is good to occasionally offer your child a choice between two acceptable, alternative foods. Sometimes he, like you, would prefer carrots to green beans. Use plates, cups, and silverware that are child-sized. Let your toddler feed himself. If he is very tired, he may need some help. Don't rush him—plan so that he has at least 20 to 30 minutes. A hurried meal cannot be pleasant.

Although you should be consistent in how you expect your child to behave at mealtimes (and at other times as well), the most important thing for you to do is maintain a calm attitude toward the whole feeding situation. Remember also to smile and hang on to your sense of humor. A good rule to follow is to couple a smile with every spoonful or forkful.

Consider each meal as part of a long chain of experiences that will help to form positive attitudes about food. Then you will appreciate that each individual success or failure is not as important as is evidence of general progress toward mature eating behavior.

Q *My toddler wants to feed himself. How can I help so he won't make such a mess?*

Toddlers may still be making a mess when they eat even though they have been feeding themselves for several months. Although some spills, missed mouthfuls, and mere playing with food are unavoidable, you can do some things to minimize these "accidents" and also to make cleaning up easier.

Toddlers often are given only spoons to eat with. This is

because parents may feel that the points on a fork are dangerous. Child-sized forks are made with a short handle and have safer, rounded tines that allow your child to spear food, which is much easier for the toddler than spooning it up.

You can also use a plastic one-cup measure filled up to ¼ cup with milk so that your toddler can easily pour out his own milk for cereal and drinking. Then he can help himself with little chance of a spill. Always choose sturdy, broad-bottomed drinking glasses that won't tip easily. Plates with rims are easier to eat from, as your toddler can push his spoon against the rim. Juicy and diced vegetables and fruits are easier to eat when served in individual custard cups or sauce dishes.

After you have done all you can to reduce the mess, try to arrange things so cleanup will be easier. Use a plastic or disposable paper place mat under your toddler's place setting. If you have a rug under the dining room table, protect the area near your child with a clear plastic cleaner's bag, or use a rubber shower mat. One day soon you'll find the place mat spotless as your child becomes more expert at feeding himself.

Q   *What should I do if my child prefers to play with his food rather than eat it?*

Grin and bear it. Part of the way that children learn about food is by touching, smelling, and smearing it. A pea can be smeared, an apple cracks, potatoes smell, and macaroni wiggles. These textural experiences are necessary to your toddler's development.

Children between the ages of one and two frequently touch, smell, and examine food before they eat it. Let your child explore within reason. Rolling peas across the high chair tray is harmless as is breaking every cracker he eats. If play gets too messy, the food should be cleared away. Sometimes children play with food when they are given large portions. It is wiser to give several small portions. This usually results in less messy play and more eating.

Q *We have occasional guests for meals. What should I expect in the way of good table manners from my two-year-old?*

Children learn good table manners by imitating the adults that they see. In that way, with a little prompting, children learn to behave in a considerate way that is the basis for good manners. Unfamiliar people at mealtime may be a strain on the child, particularly if a lot of attention is focused on him. It is better not to pay too much attention to the child or insist that he interact with the guests.

If the child remains seated, is not very noisy, and is not disrupting the others at the table, you have a well-mannered two-year-old. It is best to allow your toddler to leave the table when he has finished eating. It really is too much to expect the child to continue to sit quietly after his appetite has been satisfied.

Q *Is it a good idea to withhold foods as a punishment for a two-year-old?*

Disciplining children is a tough job. Little children at times can be frustrating, and withholding television, food, or a toy may be a simple way to get the child to obey. Although we are not experts in child behavior, we are knowledgeable about food and without a doubt we can say *never withhold food as a punishment*. For a young child, eating regularly is very important. A hungry child is grouchy and irritable. By punishing a child through food you will only wind up with a disobedient, grouchy, irritable child. In the end, you will discover that *you* are being punished more than the child.

MEALTIME SUGGESTIONS

Q *Should I still be using infant cereal for my toddler's breakfast?*

Dry instant infant cereals—rice, barley, oatmeal, mixed cereal, and high protein—are convenient to use and an economical source of many nutrients. Infant cereal is especially valuable as a source of iron. A half-ounce (4 tablespoons) serving provides your toddler with more than half of his iron requirement for the day. Regular cooked cereal, such as oatmeal, is less expensive but doesn't provide as much iron per serving.

Are you concerned that infant cereal is too much like strained infant food and not providing your toddler with enough flavor and texture? If you are, add some diced banana, diced canned fruit, grated apple, or chunky applesauce. To liven up the flavor, add some wheat germ or finely ground nuts—a teaspoon of either is enough for a serving.

Q *Any suggestions for those evenings when our 15-month-old can't eat our family dinner?*

There are many quick and easy ideas that can make a nutritious dinner for your toddler. Try these suggestions: cooked cereal; a scrambled egg; open-face toasted cheese; cottage cheese, and fruit. Most of these can be served with the dinner vegetable or with applesauce or fresh fruit and a half slice of bread to round out the meal.

Another quick idea is a variation of an Italian pasta dish that we call *Quick Noodle Casserole*.

¼ cup noodles or small-shaped pasta
1 egg, beaten
1 tablespoon grated cheese (optional)

Bring 2 cups of water to a boil; add noodles or pasta and cook according to package directions. Drain noodles or pasta into a small bowl; do not rinse; immediately pour beaten egg and cheese over noodles and toss to combine thoroughly. The heat of the pasta will cook the egg, which in turn will thicken and coat pasta mixture. Serve. Makes 2 servings, each approximately ⅓ cup.

A white sauce will serve as a meal base and can be used to combine rice, pasta, or noodles with cheese, vegetables, or shredded meat. A cooked white sauce will keep in the refrigerator up to four days, so that you can use it in small quantities as needed.

White (Cream) Sauce

Yield: 1 cup

2 tablespoons butter or margarine
2 tablespoons flour
1 cup milk

Melt butter or margarine in a small saucepan; stir in flour. Add milk slowly, continue to cook, stirring constantly until mixture thickens and boils 1 minute.

Creamed Dinner

Yield: Approximately ⅓ cup or 1 serving

¼ cup White Sauce
2 tablespoons shredded meat or flaked fish
2–3 tablespoons diced vegetable

Combine all ingredients, warm, and serve.

Quick Macaroni and Cheese

Yield: Approximately ½ cup or 1 serving

¼ cup elbow macaroni or small-shaped pasta
¼ cup White Sauce
2 tablespoons grated cheddar cheese

Cook macaroni according to package directions, drain macaroni into a small bowl; *do not* rinse. Immediately add White Sauce and cheese; stir to combine (heat of macaroni is enough to warm sauce and melt cheese). Serve.

Creamy Rice

Yield: Approximately ½ cup or 1 serving

⅓ cup cooked brown rice (white enriched rice may be substituted)
2 tablespoons peas
2 tablespoons diced carrots
¼ cup White Sauce

Combine all ingredients; warm, serve.

Creamed Soup

Yield: ¾ cup or 1 serving

¼ cup White Sauce
¼ cup milk
¼ cup diced vegetables

Combine all ingredients; warm, serve.

Q *I see baby food in my supermarket labeled "chunky" food. What is it and should I be using it?*

What you are seeing at the supermarket are toddler meals produced by Gerber* and intended for use with children one

---

* Gerber Products Co., Fremont, Michigan 49412.

to four years of age. Six meals are available: Beef and Egg Noodles, Noodles and Chicken, Vegetables and Beef, Vegetables and Chicken, Vegetables and Ham, and Vegetables and Turkey. One serving or one jar contains an average of 120 calories and the equivalent of 1 ounce serving of protein along with other needed nutrients. Combining a toddler meal with a ½ glass of milk, ½ slice of bread, and a serving of fruit for dessert provides a good meal for your child. This variety of commercial baby food is more flavorful and chunkier in consistency than strained and junior foods.

You most certainly could serve these meals to your toddler on occasion with assurance. However, they are not essential to a good diet and should not be relied on exclusively. By the time your child is a toddler he can eat most family dinnertime selections. Commercial toddler meals might be used to provide a quick lunch or dinner. Only you can judge the convenience they provide to you.

FOOD DISLIKES

Q *My child doesn't like to eat meat. How can I be sure he is getting the protein he needs?*

Many toddlers do not eat much meat; we have heard this from many mothers. It may be because meat requires more chewing than other foods. Keep offering well-cooked, ground, or other tender meats and your child may begin to enjoy it. In the meantime, there really is no need to worry about your toddler missing out on the protein he needs because other foods provide protein too. Milk, cheese, yogurt, peanut butter, and eggs are outstanding protein foods but other foods like bread, cereal, pasta, and even vegetables contain some protein.

Your toddler needs approximately 23 grams of protein

daily—that's about 2 tablespoons of pure protein. He can easily get that amount if he has 2 cups of milk (16 grams protein), plus 3 to 4 slices of bread (6 to 8 grams protein), combined with an egg (7 grams) and ½ cup of vegetables (2 grams). This totals 30 to 32 grams, which is well over the amount recommended even without eating any meat.

It is better not to make an issue of a child's refusal of a specific food; just be sure you are providing substitutes and continue to offer meat to your child and one day he'll surprise you by eating it.

Q *My toddler won't eat any cooked vegetables. How can I get him to eat some?*

Sometimes serving vegetables in an unfamiliar form such as creamed instead of plain or in matchstick pieces instead of diced may entice your child to try some. Try "new" vegetables such as bean sprouts or sliced raw kohlrabi. Offer lightly cooked or raw vegetables along with a small bowl of yogurt or creamed cottage cheese so your toddler can dip his vegetables. It also may help to serve raw vegetables at the start of a meal when your toddler is hungriest. He may be so eager to eat then that the crisp celery or carrot sticks will taste delicious. Using vegetables as a snack spread with peanut butter or cream cheese may be inviting.

Some fruits like peaches and apricots have many of the same nutrients as vegetables. Serve more of these along with cereal, eggs, bread, and meat while your toddler is acquiring a taste for vegetables. What's wrong with a dinner of mashed potatoes, peaches, and meat loaf?

Q *My 18-month-old doesn't like to drink milk. How can I encourage her to drink more?*

It isn't necessary for your child to drink all her milk; she can eat it in many other foods like cream soups (tomato, potato, and split pea are tasty), custards (both baked and boiled), milk puddings, and ice cream. Of course the puddings and ice cream usually are made with a lot of sugar so they would be appropriate only as dessert or occasional snacks. Cheese of all types are concentrated sources of milk: 1 ounce of cheddar, Swiss, or American cheese is equal to ¾ cup milk and ½ cup cottage cheese is equal to ¼ cup of milk. Remember, cream cheese is very high in fat and should be considered a spread like butter, not a milk substitute. Some children enjoy yogurt—use the unflavored type and add some fruit yourself so that it won't be as sweet as the fruit-flavored kind.

A small amount of chocolate or maple syrup added to milk may interest your toddler but be sure to add only a small amount of flavoring—1 teaspoon to ¾ cup milk—and reserve this flavored milk for one special time during the day, such as a 3 P.M. snack.

Q *Isn't it bad to give your children chocolate milk? I have heard that the chocolate does something to the calcium in the milk.*

It is true that cocoa contains a substance, oxalic acid, that combines chemically with the calcium in the milk. The complex formed prevents absorption of the calcium. Recent studies, however, have been reassuring in that they show that the small amounts of cocoa used to flavor milk would have little affect on the calcium in the milk. We recommend against children drinking only chocolate milk, but an occasional glass now and then can be a nice treat.

SNACKING

Q *My two-year-old likes to eat between meals. Is this bad for him?*

Eating between meals has become a way of life. Many of us tend to snack frequently and have only one or perhaps two regular full meals each day. What is important is the total amount of and kinds of foods that are eaten and not when they are eaten.

Small children tend to get along better with some routine in their daily activities. That's why the framework of daily meals supplemented by small snacks during the day is best. When you follow this plan it is easier to be sure that your toddler is getting all the necessary foods and also that there will not be too long a time span between eating.

You should be careful, however, that your child doesn't eat so much food in his snacks that he won't be hungry when mealtime comes around. Also, snacks should be chosen so that they will add needed nutrients, not just more sugar, salt, and fat. (See the question, "What are good snacks for a toddler?" [below].

Q *What are good snacks for a toddler?*

Chunks of fresh fruits like apples, oranges, pears, and bananas are wonderful snacks. So are other fruits and vegetables both raw and cooked. Other good choices are half slices of whole grain breads, small cubes of cheese, unsalted crackers, fruits, vegetable juices, and small servings of custard or milk pudding. Save cookies, ice cream, salted pretzels, and snack chips for occasional use.

Peanut butter is dry and sticky and may be hard for your toddler to handle. Try mixing it with a little honey or applesauce so that it will be easier to eat. A spoonful of this mixture (your toddler can eat it right off the spoon) makes a good snack with some milk or juice. Another way to use the peanut butter mixture is to dip a spoonful into crushed cereal, making a crunchy "lollipop."

Spoon-sized shredded wheat can be browned in a little melted butter in a saucepan. This tasty snack is reminiscent of popcorn and tastes just as good if not better.

Cubes of cheese skewered on pretzel sticks and cheese melted on unsalted crackers are other suggestions to try.

Q *My two-year-old will eat nothing but peanut butter and jelly sandwiches. How can I get him to eat something else?*

What you are describing is a food jag, which is perfectly normal and even expected in toddlers. Cheerfully go along with this, within reason. Allow your toddler his favorite peanut butter and jelly sandwich for lunch everyday, but offer other foods at breakfast and dinner. Don't be surprised if at first the other foods are refused. Be patient, as after a meal or two hunger will win out. Your child will quickly realize that every lunch meal will be his prized peanut butter and jelly, and he should accept other foods at breakfast and dinner. Be prepared, however, for the day he'll suddenly reject peanut butter and jelly and fall in love with toasted cheese!

Q *My neighbor's child is always "nibbling" on meat sticks. Should I be giving these to my child?*

You could. The product is available in the baby food aisle of your supermarket packed in 2½-ounce glass jars. Chicken, turkey, and meat sticks (a combination of pork, beef, and turkey) provide approximately seven 2-inch sticks per container. They are a protein-rich snack or can be used for a meal. A serving of 3½ meat sticks equals 7.5 grams of protein or about the equivalent of 1 ounce of meat, fish, or poultry. Lower in fat and free of the additives and preservatives normally found in hot dogs or luncheon meat, meat sticks are a good substitute for these foods for your toddler. However, you should realize that if meat sticks are unit-priced they cost over $3.50 a pound.

Q *What's the difference between "toddler pretzels" and regular pretzels?*

"Toddler pretzels" are available in the infant food section of the supermarket. Nutritionally they are the same as regular pretzels, however toddler pretzels are lower in sodium (salt) but more costly per ounce.

Regardless of what type you buy, don't hand them out liberally to your toddler. We've seen small children who walk around most of the day *eating,* a bad habit.

Q *Which is better, cookies made specifically for toddlers or regular cookies?*

Too many of *any* type of cookie is not good for your child. Handed out in moderation, plain cookies, whether made specifically for the toddler or not, are fine as an occasional snack or dessert. Below is a chart giving you the protein, fat, carbohydrate, and caloric value of cookies. As you can see, the ones produced by commercial baby food companies and the ones produced by cookie manufacturers do not differ a great deal. All of the cookies listed could be given to a toddler. Your child, like all children, will enjoy cookies because they taste good and allow him to feed himself.

Cookie	Serving	Calories per serving	Protein, g	Fat, g	Carbohydrate, g	Cost per ounce, ¢
Arrowroot cookies (Gerber)	2 cookies	50	1.0	2.0	8.0	16
Arrowroot cookies (Nabisco)	2 cookies	42	0.86	1.06	7.22	12
Animal crackers (Nabisco, Barnum's)	3 cookies	27	0.36	0.57	4.74	25
Animal cookies (Gerber)	2 cookies	60	2.0	2.0	9.0	14
Fig Newton	1 piece	55	0.45	0.99	10.9	10
Graham (Nabisco)	1 cracker	30	0.52	0.74	5.35	9
Lorna Doone (Nabisco)	1 cookie	38	0.56	1.66	5.14	14
Oatmeal cookie (Nabisco)	1 cookie	86	1.32	3.06	13.2	10
Ritz cracker	1 cracker	17	0.24	0.87	2.0	9
Saltine	1 cracker	14	0.29	0.38	2.32	5
Waverly wafers	1 wafer	18	0.27	0.80	2.52	9
Zwiebach	1 piece	31	0.87	0.67	5.43	22
Zwiebach (Gerber)	1 piece	30	0.5	1.0	5.0	17

POOR APPETITE

Q *My two-year-old is eating less; sometimes he refuses all food. What can I do?*

Most two-year-old children become less interested in food because they are no longer growing rapidly; growth requires a great deal of energy. Though he may seem more active than ever, he eats less.

If you become upset about your toddler's refusal to eat, that may make the situation worse. It's fun for your child to have the attention and fuss that happens when he doesn't eat.

At mealtimes simply serve the food with no comment. After 20 minutes or so, remove all uneaten food, again with no comment. Don't be concerned that your child will starve; he won't. He might ask for some food an hour or so after mealtime. When he does give him a small amount of juice or milk and a cracker or small serving of fruit. Don't offer a large snack thinking he is *very* hungry since he ate so little at the last meal. You want snacks to complement a meal, not substitute for one. A small snack will insure that he will be hungry at the next regular mealtime.

Don't be surprised if your child refuses a number of meals in a row. This is often a test of his independence. Remove the uneaten meal, with no comment; offer a *small* snack if requested. You may have to do this several times. Remain calm; when your child is hungry he will eat. If his refusal to eat persists, check with the doctor to be sure that he is well and that his height and weight gain is normal for his age. If he is doing well, relax! To help interest your toddler in eating be sure to serve small portions, serve the food attractively, and try some new interesting foods occasionally.

Q *My neighbor's toddler is a very poor eater. Won't this have a long-range effect on his development?*

"Poor eater" is a general term that can mean anything from a finicky eater to a child who truly eats too little or eats very poor food choices.

A fussy or finicky eater may be difficult to satisfy but in almost all cases the child eats enough food, within a narrow range of selections, to support growth and development. A daily vitamin/mineral supplement might insure that this child gets a good daily complement of nutrients as a supplement to round out his food. Most children who are finicky eaters mature into adventurous adults. (See the question, "How do you feed a finicky eater?" on page 38.) A child who is fed very poor selections, or too little food, may suffer long-term effects. We once counseled a young mother who fed her toddler son a diet that consisted mostly of chocolate milk, canned spaghetti, and M&M candies. Not only were the food selections poor but the amounts given were so small that the boy's growth was already slow for his age. Recently an international team of investigators found that poor diet in children can be linked to emotional instability. They observed that toddlers who were underfed were more likely to have reduced sociability, lack of interest in their environment, and inadequate emotional development by school age. The results suggest that poor nutrition, which can result in subtle alterations in normal development, often combines with a poor home environment to stunt a child's potential emotional well-being. See the question, "Since my child began nursery school she refuses to eat dinner. What can I do?" on page 42.

HEALTH CONCERNS

Q *My neighbor says my toddler looks pale. Could she be anemic?*

You really cannot tell if children are anemic by their skin color alone. Many children normally have a pale skin tone. The way to find out is by a simple blood test your doctor can do. This blood test is done routinely at the 6- and 18-month checkups and may also be done at 12 and 24 months. If you are concerned about anemia, ask your doctor to do a blood test.

Q *My 20-month-old looks very chubby. What type of diet can I put him on?*

It's not a good idea to put a toddler on a reducing diet, as it really isn't necessary for him to lose weight. A better idea is to limit further weight gain and let nature take its course and wait for your child to grow into his weight. Simple adjustments you can make are to eliminate sweets, soda, and salty snacks. Use fruits and vegetables for snacks and when your toddler is thirsty, give him water to drink. Although skim milk is not advised for children under age two, you might try some low-fat, 2-percent milk if it is available in your area. This has a little less fat and calories than regular whole milk and it is well liked by children.

Try to increase your child's activity. See that he is outside playing actively for at least half an hour each morning and afternoon. A brisk walk around the block will be good for both of you. What is a moderate pace for you will be a trot for the toddler.

The chubby toddler is best treated with a moderate approach, more activity, and fewer sugary, salty, high-fat snacks. In a few months you'll be pleased to see your boy slimming out as he grows a little and maintains his weight. See Chapter 7 for more information on handling an overweight child.

LEAD POISONING

Q *My child eats cigarette butts whenever he gets the chance, is this dangerous?*

In our experience counseling, we have seen children who routinely ate comics, cigarettes, paint chips, dirt, rug lint, crayons, and other odd substances. All of these children, as well as your child, display pica: the eating of nonfood substances.

What causes this behavior? We don't know. The desire in some children is for a single food, such as ice, crackers, pretzels, pickles, potato chips, and some vegetables. One preschool boy reportedly ate a "large" jar of pickles daily. Reports of dirt, clay, and charcoal eating date back to A.D. 1,000.

Pica in small children is often the result of normal curiosity; almost anything they touch goes in their mouth. Your child may be eating cigarettes to mimic your smoking. You place the cigarette in your mouth and the child perceives this as "eating." Keep cigarettes away from your child and discuss the problem with your doctor if it persists. Most young children naturally stop these habits once their curiosity is satisfied but for a few, pica can be harmful.

Many nonfood items such as starch, dirt, paint, and cigarettes, contain substances, like lead, that can cause illness or poisoning. (See the following question, "How do children get lead poisoning?" for more information.) Anemia may also be a symptom of pica. Clay and ice eaters often are anemic.

Q *How do children get lead poisoning?*

All children are exposed to some lead each day in air, water, and household dust. Lead poisoning occurs after a child has accidentally consumed too much lead. Toddlers often "eat" anything available—peeling paint or plaster, makeup (especially eyeliner and eyeshadow), cigarettes, colored newsprint—all containing lead. Ceramic pottery, particularly the type imported from Mexico and South America, is often glazed with lead-based paint. Pewter made into cups and food containers is an alloy of tin, lead, and other metals. Old water pipes and heavy auto traffic further increase exposure. (Water pipes in newer homes are lead free).

If a toddler has a heavy exposure to lead, the levels of this metal in the body become excessively high and lead poisoning or intoxication results. This can cause anemia, behavior changes, and in severe cases brain damage or even death. A blood test will determine lead levels. If you feel your child has had excessive exposure to lead he should be tested.

A reassuring note: In the early-1970s formula, infant juices and evaporated milk were the major sources of lead in a toddler's diet because these foods were in contact with the lead solder used to seal the cans. Replacement of these cans with jars (juices) and the redesign of the formula can so it is unsoldered eliminated the risk. Evaporated milk is still packaged in a lead-soldered can and therefore should not be used as the major milk source for a toddler.

Q *Is it true that canned juices are poisonous?*

Recently, a few cases of lead poisoning in children were traced to fruit juice stored in open cans. One 8-ounce glass of the juice these children drank contained the maximum allowable daily level of lead for young children. The lead in the juice came from migration of lead from the soldered seams of the can.

After opening canned juice, contact with air speeds up the leeching of lead from the solder into the juice. The longer fruit juice is stored in an open can, the more likely it is that lead will be found in the juice. We would recommend buying juice packaged in bottles or cardboard containers. If canned juice is bought, after opening it should be stored in a nonmetallic container.

TODDLER QUIZ

Now that we have answered some of your questions, we would like to ask you some questions so you can assess how well you are feeding your child.

Your toddler usually:	Yes	No
has meals or snacks four or more times a day.	☐	☐
is served food with no comment.	☐	☐
is given "toddler-sized" portions.	☐	☐
is served a new food at the beginning of a meal, when his appetite is greatest.	☐	☐
is not hurried to finish eating.	☐	☐
eats in a quiet, pleasant setting.	☐	☐
is occasionally given choices between two acceptable alternatives.	☐	☐
is served snack foods low in sugar and salt and fat.	☐	☐
is usually encouraged to feed himself.	☐	☐
is offered foods from each of the four food groups at each meal.	☐	☐
is offered food from each of two food groups at a snacktime.	☐	☐

Two

Preschool Nutrition (Ages 4 to 6)

> *"A child must touch, feel,*
> *see, taste, smell, hear, and*
> *. . . spill a little milk in*
> *order to grow."**

Spilling milk may be one of the most common characteristics of children aged four to six. There was a time in Laura's life when she spilled a glassful every day. When Karen was small, the family motto was "only pour as much as you want to wipe up." Wiggling, fidgeting, and talking incessantly is typical of preschoolers. Put this all together and you will eat many meals on a soggy tablecloth, with a jumping jack, answering so many questions you'll barely have time to chew!

At the preschool age children are broadening their experiences and learning rapidly. They become fiercely independent, wanting to serve themselves one day and steadfastly refusing to eat the next. Appetite fluctuations and strange

---

* From a poster by Growing Child, P.O. Box 620, Lafayette, Indiana 47902.

food combinations, though unnerving, are common. After toddlerhood and before first grade children are in a "thinning out" period—growing in height with a very slow growth in weight. They may eat *very* small amounts of food, and judging by adult portions, you are convinced your child is starving. This "starving" child, however, is the picture of health, with boundless energy. Young children are reliable judges of how much they need to eat. Left on their own, with no urging or coaxing, they will eat to appetite—eating when hungry, stopping when full. That's a habit many adults wish they had. Parents, however, with the best intentions, sabotage this natural appetite control by offering too much food and insisting on "clean plates" or worst yet "happy plates." This tells the child loud and clear that an "unhappy plate" (full) is bad. At this age a child and his actions are one and the same. A bad act, in the child's mind, makes him a bad person. Eating a certain food in a certain way has little to do with being "good" or "bad." Yet numerous adults automatically classify food as "good-for-you" or "bad-for-you," and feel either virtuous or guilty for what they have eaten.

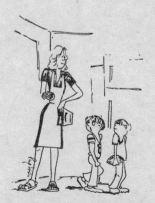

No, thank you, Mrs. Johnson,
I don't eat broken cookies.

MY FAVORITE MEAL

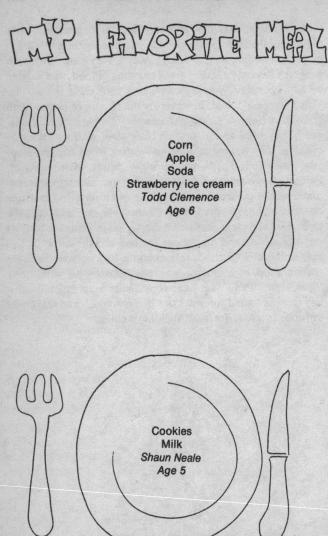

Corn
Apple
Soda
Strawberry ice cream
Todd Clemence
Age 6

Cookies
Milk
Shaun Neale
Age 5

Ages three to six are special years for your child's nutritional development. During these years, for perhaps the last time, you still have almost total control over what your child eats. At this age children of all cultures form their ideas about food—what is edible, poisonous, neutral, taboo, and disgusting. The opinions and attitudes they form will influence food consumption for the rest of their lives.

Q *How do you get a child to eat what's good for him?*

That's a simple question that doesn't have a simple answer. It is important, however, to make an effort to get children to eat nutritious food. Studies show that food patterns and attitudes established during the preschool years affect food choices and nutrition status throughout life. Good habits formed at this stage can lay the foundation for good health.

Here are a few basic eating principles you might try:

* *Don't use food as a pacifier, reward, or punishment.* These gimmicks bestow on food an emotional value that may outweigh nutritional considerations.

* *Don't worry about how little a child eats.* The average child increases his weight 300 percent in the first year of life but only 12 percent a year between three and five. This slow growth needs less food to support it. If your child's growth rate is normal he is eating enough.

* *Set a good example.* A young child is a reflection of his parents. If you eat erratically and make poor food choices how can you expect your child to do otherwise? A survey showed that vegetable likes and dislikes of young children were directly related to the father's likes and dislikes.

* *Limit the amount of less desirable foods kept in the house.* Children will happily eat cakes, cookies, candy, and soda if they are made readily available. Stock your

Daily Food Guide for the Preschool Child

A preschool child needs daily:

Milk
 2 cups
 1 serving = ½ cup

Use whole milk, evaporated milk (reconstituted with water), skim milk, nonfat dry milk, buttermilk, cheese, yogurt.

Meat, Fish, Poultry, and Protein-Rich Foods
 3 servings
 1 serving = 1 ounce*

Egg, cheese, dried peas or beans, tofu, peanut, or other nut butters may be substituted for a serving of meat, fish, or poultry.

Vegetables and Fruit
 4 or more servings
 1 serving of vegetable = ¼ cup
 1 serving of fruit   = 1 small fresh fruit
         = ¼ cup cooked or canned fruit

1 serving of a vitamin C–rich food (orange, grapefruit, melon, strawberries, broccoli, tomatoes, coleslaw). 1 serving of a vitamin A–rich food, dark green or deep yellow-orange in color (spinach, sweet potato, carrot, apricot, and mango).
2 or more servings of other fruits and vegetables (including potatoes).

Bread, Cereal, Rice, Pasta
 3 to 4 servings
 1 serving = ½ slice bread
      = ¼ cup cooked cereal, pasta, or rice
      = ⅓–½ cup dry cereal

Use only whole grain and enriched products.

* See page 7 for portion sizes of 1 ounce of protein.

house, instead, with fruit juice, fresh fruit, nuts, yogurt, popcorn, and other more desirable foods.

- *Make your own treats.* When making your own cakes and cookies you can control the amount of sugar and fat used. In addition, you can include whole grains, nuts, and fruits. Letting your child help you make treats almost guarantees he'll eat them.

- *Don't be afraid to set limits.* If your child is clamoring for a food you feel is not good, say "No, I want you to drink milk or juice, not soda. You need milk for healthy bones." Counter the propaganda a child sees and hears with facts.

MEALTIME BEHAVIOR

Q *My four-year-old daughter insists I set a place for her imaginary friend at every meal. Should I?*

Most definitely, yes. Part of the joy of being four years old is the fun of having your own imaginary friend. One of our children had an imaginary "monk-me" (monkey) who regularly ate with the family.

Often you can use the imaginary friend to get a child to try new food. "Kristen, did you know that your "monk-me" told me he'd like to try a little cauliflower? Would you like to try some too?" Preoccupation with sharing a meal with the imaginary friend may keep the child interested in eating for a longer time and less apt to get restless and fidgety.

Most imaginary friends don't get much older than four, so by the time your daughter turns five she'll find her old friend is too young to play with and she'll stop bringing him to dinner.

Q *Why does my four-year-old child announce he must go to the bathroom in the middle of every meal?*

Four-year-olds have many predictable traits—a bathroom visit during each meal is very common. Children this age are beginning to become more engrossed in activities. Rather than disturb what they are doing, they ignore the urge to go to the bathroom. Meals often interrupt this intense activity. After a few minutes of eating, during which time the entire digestive tract is stimulated, the urge returns, at times so intensely that a trip to the bathroom becomes an emergency.

Knowing this is normal, when you call your son to eat, remind him to wash his hands *and* go to the bathroom before he sits down at the table. This will usually eliminate the mid meal scramble to the bathroom.

Q *My husband gets annoyed because our five-year-old has terrible table manners. What should I do?*

When good manners are placed above a pleasant family meal, tension builds and tempers flare. Eating should be relaxed and natural with as few artificial rules as possible. Good manners evolve, sometimes very slowly, by imitating parents and older siblings. If you or older children are poor models you can't expect your five-year-old to act like "Emily Post."

A five-year-old who has made progress eating quietly; is able to use a knife, fork, and spoon; resorts to fingers only occasionally; seldom upsets his drink; uses a napkin; and on occasion says "please" and "thank you" spontaneously is well mannered. Regimenting dinner behavior results in a child who is not likely to enjoy meals.

Some trouble spots can be avoided with a little forethought. Make sure the child can comfortably reach the table. Using a higher chair or pillow makes reaching the table easier. Try eating your own meal with your chin barely above the table and your arms at shoulder height and see how neat you are. A cobbler's apron or painter's smock can protect the child's clothing so you don't need a bib. Precut or fix the child's portion to facilitate eating. If you cut spaghetti into manageable pieces, father is less likely to get annoyed watching a red strand dangling against the child's shirt. Even when a fork is provided many children prefer to "scoop" with a spoon. Don't insist on a fork. If dinner is long (anything over 10 minutes is long to a five-year-old) excuse the child to play quietly after he's finished his main course and call him back to join the family for dessert.

A patient, flexible attitude about eating is the only sensible approach to take. Otherwise, family meals become battlefields where no one enjoys the food.

Q *Should a child who doesn't finish his meal be given dessert?*

We like to think of dessert as a part of the whole meal rather than a reward for a clean plate. How many times have you heard "No dessert until you eat every bite on your plate." This implies that desserts are a better part of the meal, a prize you receive after you suffer through the task of eating. How inappropriate! This puts undue emphasis on desserts and makes them very desirable to a child.

When offered as dessert, pudding, custard, yogurt, fruit, even ice cream, contribute many essential nutrients to a meal. Regardless of how much or how little the child eats, allow him to have dessert. Remember, though, dessert is not supposed to make up for a meal the child refused to eat or to finish. Offer only one serving of the dessert you planned. If the child asks for more, simply say one dessert is enough and suggest eating more dinner if he is still hungry.

Children constantly test parents to discover their boundaries. Knowing his boundaries adds to his feelings of security. Trying to get dessert without eating dinner may be a test. You establish boundaries by limiting the quantity of dessert offered so he could not possibly be filled by one serving. The time the food is eaten during the meal is not really important. Kristen, who loved pudding, always ate it along with her meal because she could not stand to wait till the main course was over. Often her meal flavor combinations were quite strange—macaroni and cheese, tossed salad, plus butterscotch pudding. Once she realized, however, that we were not going to withhold the pudding and we didn't care when she ate it, pudding once again ended the meal rather than being a feature of the main course.

TROUBLE SPOTS

Q *How do you feed a finicky eater?*

There was a time when Kristen lived on breakfast cereal, toast, and raisins washed down with large amounts of grape juice. Having a dietitian for a mother, it seemed inconceivable that no matter how hard she was coaxed to "just take one bite" her diet remained unchanged by all assaults.

As hard as we tried, her eating habits were often a source of tension in the house. At times we were frustrated—"If she'd only try . . ." Sometimes we ignored the situation—"What she eats is her business." And sometimes we were angry—"If she doesn't eat what's on the table she can just go hungry!" None of these approaches worked until we started using the advice that I confidently gave other families:

Accept the fact that some children are finicky and no amount of threats, coercion, or rewards will get them to try a food that does not appeal to them. Children forced to eat a food that repels them may establish a food aversion that could last most of their lives.

Ask your child to tell you all the foods he likes. Flip through a magazine and have him pick out things he'd eat. Make a list of them. Kristen selected from food models used to counsel patients and surprisingly her selections were reasonably varied. Then we set up a system of acceptable substitutes for dinner items that did not involve cooking a second meal. The rule for meals was simple: at each meal you must eat three different foods.

Bread, noodles, rice, pasta, and potatoes were considered as one group and were usually an acceptable choice to the child. Contrary to popular opinion children don't like creamed foods, sauces, or casseroles. They love noodles, rice, potatoes, and pasta plain. Hold some out of the more seasoned dish you are preparing and restrain yourself from commenting about how uninteresting the plain version is. Young children often refuse to eat meat. Don't despair, as there are many other sources of protein to substitute. We kept hard-cooked eggs in the refrigerator or a slice of cheese; or offered a dollop of peanut butter or a handful of nuts. These substitutes required no additional cooking while adding a good protein source to the meal. Vegetables are always troublesome so we allowed for a fresh fruit substitution or reserved a raw portion of the family selection. Children who hate cooked vegetables will often eat raw celery, carrots, and peppers.

Some of Kristen's dinners looked strange: meat loaf, baked potato, and a banana; rice, nuts, and raw carrots; plain spaghetti, peanut butter on Italian bread sticks, and an apple. Not exactly gourmet fare but reasonably varied and balanced. Each meal was accompanied by juice or milk.

Q How can I get my child to try a new food?

Neophobia, fear of something new, is a definite factor that limits the types of food a child will eat. As a child grows and matures, new things become challenging rather than fearsome and all experiences, including food choices, broaden. Generally, the more a child is exposed to a particular food, even if he doesn't eat it, the more neutral his feelings about the food become. This is known as *habituation.* Once the emotional response to a food is lessened, the child will usually try it and judge it on its own merits. Children begin to become more adventurous, willingly tasting new foods, between ages seven and nine. Be patient and in a few years you'll see a difference.

Q What's wrong with my 4½-year-old daughter who has very little appetite?

One of the most frequent complaints we hear from parents of preschoolers is that their child has no appetite. In most cases, what the parents perceive as "no appetite" is simply a slowing down or lessened appetite resulting from a slower growth at this age. As long as the child is growing, even slowly, and is healthy, there is nothing to worry about. Some children are naturally small and thin with small appetites. Don't cajole or coerce the child to eat, since these efforts may result in mealtimes becoming a tug-of-war between the parent and child. The Daily Food Guide for the Preschooler, page 34, will help you to see how much your child should eat each day. You might be surprised to find it's less than you realized or less than you are expecting your daughter to eat. Also appreciate that a small child can't eat much at one meal. Many children between the ages of three and five need to eat six times a day—three small meals with a midmorning, midafternoon, and bedtime snack.

Q   *What's wrong with my five-year-old who is irritable and cranky in hot weather and has no appetite?*

Your child is perfectly normal. During the summer our appetites may wane while our desire for fluids increases markedly. This is particularly true of children, therefore, don't force them to eat. Breakfast and an evening snack may be the best times to offer food. A fruit bowl can satisfy midday hunger if lunch is light or skipped completely.

The summer heat causes loss of body fluids so that we are naturally more thirsty. This is especially true of young children who cannot reach the water faucet or get into the refrigerator easily. When children are mildly dehydrated they become irritable and lack energy. A picnic thermos can be filled each day and left in a convenient spot where even the smallest child can serve himself when thirsty.

Avoid excessively sweetened drink mixes since they are long on calories and short on nutrients. Stick with unsweetened fruit juices and don't overlook simple cold water—it's refreshing. An excellent summer soda, which is additive- and sugar-free, is one part fruit juice mixed with one part club soda. It's effervescent, cool, and nutritious. Add a few ice cubes for fun.

During the summer your child will eat more fresh fruits and vegetables. However, due to the widespread use of insecticides, herbicides, and fungicides on crops, remember to *wash* all fresh fruit before eating it. Rinsing under running water removes only about 20 percent of the pesticide residue on food. A more effective way to remove the residue is to wash the fruit with dilute kitchen detergent and then rinse with water. If a handbrush is used to spread the detergent over the surface, cleaning is even more thorough. Removal of the outer portions of leafy vegetables, such as cabbage and lettuce, greatly reduces pesticide intake.

Q *Since my child began nursery school she refuses to eat dinner. What can I do?*

Sudden loss of appetite or refusal to eat, by a young child, is often a reaction to change. In your case, the experience of adjusting to nursery school may be the key. Even if your child enjoys school there is a certain amount of apprehension about leaving you and coping alone in a new situation.

Loss of appetite is usually associated with a new or perhaps difficult situation that the child is facing—new school, family problems, new baby, sibling rivalry, death of a family member or friend, overprotective parent-child relationship, or problems with peers. Overstimulation may also be a cause. Too much excitement or too much activity can leave a young child too exhausted to eat. Your child may need a quiet, relaxing period or nap before dinner, if nursery school meets in the morning. Also consider the time of your usual dinner hour. Perhaps an early nursery school session has extended your child's normal waking day and dinner is now just too late. Don't make an issue of not eating since this will only prolong the problem. Try serving foods the child particularly likes or encouraging help with preparation. Both of these suggestions often result in interest in the meal. Even if the child still doesn't eat dinner offer a bedtime snack. Pick nutritious foods and keep the servings small, no seconds. This will help to make up for the missed meal but will not substitute for it. A slice of toast, dish of applesauce, cheese, and crackers are all good choices. Above all, relax, since loss of appetite in young children is usually a temporary problem.

Q *My five-year-old refuses to eat breakfast. What can I do?*

You have probably heard how necessary breakfast is to supply energy for the morning activities. What you may not realize is that whether or not people are breakfast eaters often depends on habits formed in their childhood. That is why it is a good idea to offer your child some food soon after he wakes up in the morning. In that way you are setting the stage for future breakfast eating. Why not try some different foods or even some familiar foods served in a different way to get your child more interested in breakfast? Half a grilled cheese or tuna fish sandwich with a glass of milk makes a fine breakfast, so would some cottage cheese spread on toast or crackers. Even leftovers like meat loaf are fine. Any type of nutritious wholesome food is just as good at breakfast time as it is at any other time.

Try serving your child the usual dry cereal and milk separately. A pile of Cheerios on a plate that can be easily eaten with fingers is fun. A sliced banana can be added for some interest. Add a glass of milk and you have a well-rounded breakfast.

If you are not rushed in the morning, why not let your child help you make some breakfast foods like corn muffins or cinnamon whole wheat toast. Be sure to eat along with your child, as mothers who skip breakfast often have children that do the same.

SNACKING

Q *Is it normal for a five-year-old to snack all day and not eat regular meals?*

Your child is not the least bit unusual. Young children have small stomachs and small appetites and need frequent refueling; two to four snacks a day plus meals would be a normal meal pattern. We like to refer to a child such as yours as a *grazing child*—a child who eats many times throughout the day but who rarely eats a complete meal at one sitting. The key to feeding a grazing child is to provide reasonable snack choices and stretch out some meals so that a part of the meal becomes the next snack. For example, you might plan a lunch of soup, crackers, an apple, and milk. Your child eats the soup and crackers, drinks most of the milk, takes one bite of the apple, and declares "I'm done." You coax him to eat a little more apple and finish the milk. He squirms and plays with the food till you allow him to go and play. You know your child likes apples, so why didn't he eat it? The answer is that *young children have small stomachs and small appetites and need frequent refueling.*

Here's another way to have handled the situation: plan the same lunch but serve only the soup and crackers with a juice glass full of milk. An hour or so later when your son announces, "I'm hungry," offer another small glass of milk and the apple. You have offered no more food than you normally would; you simply offered it stretched out to fit the child's natural hunger.

Well-chosen snack foods can make a positive contribution to a child's diet. Even a sweet snack provides energy (calories) and is enjoyable. Don't make your child feel guilty if he snacks on a small portion of a favorite food merely for the pleasure of it. That's eating in a rational way, something more adults should learn.

Don't feel that snacking automatically leads to obesity. On the contrary, it has been found that slender children eat more snacks, as opposed to planned meals, than their heavier counterparts. Further, the frequency of eating had no effect on the total calories consumed for a day. The grazing child seems to listen to his natural hunger drive—eating when hungry, stopping when full—an excellent habit to establish. (See the next question, "What are good between-meal snacks?")

Q *What are good between-meal snacks?*

Preschool children may snack up to four times a day, making these "minimeals" an important part of their daily food intake. The snacks this age group lists as favorites, in decreasing order of importance, are bakery products (mostly cookies), milk, soft drinks, milk desserts, candy, and bread.

Before we give you some good snack suggestions, let's define what a snack is. A snack is a small quantity of food eaten at other than mealtimes. It should never substitute for or prevent a child from eating a regular meal. A child who has enjoyed a nutritious snack 45 minutes to an hour before mealtime will still have a healthy appetite for the meal. A slice of buttered or plain whole wheat bread is a nice predinner snack that we often used with our own children to ward off the hunger pangs that made waiting for dinner intolerable.

Easy and nutritious snacks

Raw vegetables

Fresh or canned fruit

Applesauce

Fruit juice ice pops*

Dry cereal (to eat as a nibble)

Crackers and cheese

Crackers and peanut butter

Cheese cubes

Popcorn, unbuttered

Frozen banana

Yogurt

Ice cream

Annette's mandlebrot*

Whole grain bread

Bread sticks

Baldy pretzels

Create a Crunch*

Granola bars*

Yogurt shake*

Create a soda*

Half of a sandwich

Hard-cooked egg

Create a pudding*

Custard

Spread on crackers
  or bread.**

See the sections in Chapters 1, 3, and 4 on snacking to give you even more ideas.

* Recipes in Part III, Kid-Tested Recipes.
** Spread suggestions on page 92.

Q *Are frankfurters safe to eat?*

Americans eat almost 8 pounds of hot dogs per person per year. It is a food served in 95 percent of homes. Interestingly, adults eat more hot dogs than children and women eat more hot dogs than men. If it is such a popular food what could be wrong with it? Questions that are most often asked about hot dogs are: what goes into the casing and are the chemicals used harmful?

From time to time a horror story circulates that "garbage meats" or undesirable animal parts (snouts, lips, feet) are used to make hot dogs. In 1973 new USDA regulations were established for hot dog labels. All ingredients must be listed in decreasing order of quantity. Meat by-products (variety meats) and mechanically deboned meat may be used but if they are, the label must prominently say "frankfurters with by-products" or "frankfurters with mechanically processed products." Hot dogs may contain up to 15 percent poultry meat, if labeled accordingly. Up to 3½ percent nonfat dry milk, cereal, or dried whole milk or 2 percent soy protein may be added if declared on the label. These binders often increase the protein value and decrease the fat content of the traditional all-meat hot dog. Hot dogs made of all chicken, turkey, veal, or vegetable protein are also available. They may be lower in fat and calories than the regular hot dog. Their labels must also fully state their ingredients. Other ingredients often used in making hot dogs are water, sugar or dextrose, spices, and curing agents.

Sodium nitrates and nitrites, added to hot dogs to inhibit the growth of bacteria that causes botulism, a deadly food poisoning, have been opposed because of their possible link to cancer. These preservatives can combine in the stomach with amines, forming nitrosamines, which are carcinogenic (cancer-causing). It must be understood that nitrates and nitrites occur naturally in some vegetables and in saliva. Eating a food or drinking a juice high in vitamin C at the same time as you eat hot dogs helps to prevent the formation of nitrosamines. Serve your children hot dogs with orange juice.

Eating hot dogs once a week is fine. We'd discourage frequent use because of their fat and salt content. An average hot dog has approximately 125 calories, 90 of which are from fat. The hot dog has about the same fat content as lean chopped meat.

SWEETS

Q *Is it true that children have a natural desire for sweets?*

Researchers who work with newborn infants find that they show inborn preferences for sweets. They make pleased faces when given sweet-tasting liquids and drinks more of a sweeter liquid than of a less sweet liquid. We deduce from this and other taste research that there are genetically inborn likes and dislikes. These preferences, however, can be modified or enhanced through conditioning and experiences with food.

When children and adults were tested for their perception of sweetness both identified sweet-tasting foods as sweet. The children, however, continued to accept and enjoy foods that became increasingly sweeter in taste. Adults reached a point at which the sweetness became cloying and unacceptable and they disliked the food due to its sweetness. The sweet tooth of children will accept larger amounts of sugar.

In practical terms this means a mildly sweet cookie and an iced, heavily sweetened cookie will be accepted just the same by a child. The unsweetened cookie will be rejected. Therefore, we can condition children to enjoy lightly sweetened foods—put ½ teaspoon of sugar on breakfast cereal but don't offer a presweetened variety.

An interesting note on this issue: obese adults find acceptable levels of sweet tastes above what normal-weight adults identify as far too sweet for their liking.

Q *Should I buy the vitamin C–fortified lollipops I saw in the supermarket?*

Some foods are enriched with added nutrients to enhance their nutritional quality, or the food is used as a vehicle to supply a population with a needed nutrient. Vitamin D, added to milk, all but eliminated bone-deforming rickets. Adding vitamin C to lollipops, however, smacks of a marketing gimmick. This "nutritional bonus" was probably added to allay the mother's guilt and/or entice her to buy a sweet she might otherwise ignore. Surely, vitamin C–fortified lollipops won't harm your child but there are far better food sources.

Q *Which is the best candy for my child to eat?*

We think that small amounts of candy can be enjoyed as an occasional treat. For children of preschool age, candy miniatures are a good choice, in very small portions. Avoid those candies which are sticky, like caramels and gumdrops or those candies which are sucked, like sour balls or lollipops. For more information on candy see Chapter 6, Dental Health.

Q *How can I be assured that candy I buy at the supermarket has not been tampered with?*

You are obviously referring to the Tylenol scare in the fall of 1982, when seven people died after taking capsules containing cyanide. That incident made every consumer more aware. As of February 1984, all over-the-counter drug products were required by the FDA to have tamper-resistant containers. The industry prefers to call them *tamper-evident* since the design of the container will make it obvious to the consumer if someone has tried to open the package.

Food products aren't covered by FDA regulations though many companies are voluntarily introducing tamper-resistant packaging. Baby food jars have always been sealed with a lid that has a center section that pops up when the lid is opened. Unopened, the center of the lid is depressed. A decided "pop" is heard upon opening. Other jarred food items are adopting the same button-pop lid. Candy manufacturers are using a film wrap on candy trays which has an identifying logo. This wrap can't be replaced or punctured as easily as clear wrap. Other candy manufacturers have removed air holes from plastic bags of miniature bars so they are not mistaken for pinpricks.

You can teach your children to be more cautious consumers. Never encourage them to nibble from opened cookie or candy boxes found on supermarket shelves. Point out damaged packages and explain why you don't buy them. When they are helping you put food items in the cart, say "Have you checked that for cracks or holes?" Young children will enjoy this "inspector's" job and learn in the process.

One last point: despite the consumer's heightened concern for safety, food manufacturers claim the consumer is still more likely to complain about a product that is too difficult to open than about one that is too easily opened.

Q *Besides cake and ice cream, what are some good party foods to serve for my five-year-old's birthday party?*

Young children have small appetites which are easily satisfied by party food. Planning a mealtime party is a nice idea. Noontime is probably best, leaving afternoon to rest or nap after the party excitement. Mealtime parties should last one to two hours. Longer than this, the small child becomes over-stimulated and irritable, turning a good time sour. The younger the child, the fewer the guests. Six to ten children at this age is a houseful.

Simple, familiar food attractively served will be most successful. Hot dogs and buns served with fresh raw vegetables are a popular choice. Some parents may not wish to serve a processed meat. If that is so, try these menu suggestions:

Open-face toasted cheese
Apple wedges

Graham crackers spread with peanut butter topped with thinly sliced apple rounds

Ants on a log (celery stuffed with peanut butter topped with raisins)
Cheese cubes
Bread sticks

Raw green pepper rings topped with a meatball
Toasted whole wheat Italian bread

Sandwiches cut with a cookie cutter*
Celery sticks

Whole wheat waffles
Sausages
Orange sections

English-muffin pizza
Tossed salad

Create a sandwich
Dried fruit

Milk, apple cider, or fruit juice can be served with these menus. To be festive serve chocolate milk with a dollop of

* See sandwich spread ideas on page 92.

whipped cream; orange juice with cranberry-juice ice cubes; any fruit juice mixed half and half with seltzer and garnished with pineapple chunks on a skewer.

Don't omit the birthday cake, which is the highlight of the party. Ice cream cakes are not as sugary as bakery cakes. Ice a nutritious muffin and arrange all the muffins on a platter to look like a cake; divide to serve. If a traditional cake is served, keep the pieces small. An occasional sweet treat is not inappropriate, especially at a birthday party.

CEREALS

Q *Which is the best cereal to buy?*

If you listened to cereal advertisements you'd probably pick a highly sweetened, high-fiber, vitamin- and mineral-fortified cereal. You'd also be paying a premium price.

Cooked wheat, barley, or corn served as a porridge or mush were ancient, commonly used foods, served at any meal of the day. "Cold" breakfast cereals are a modern-day innovation that have their roots in the late 1800s when the Kellogg brothers invented flaked wheat and flaked corn. These "healthful" foods were served at their fashionable sanatorium in Battle Creek, Michigan. One of the Kellogg followers was a man named C. W. Post, who invented Grape-Nuts. In each box of cereal, Post included a nutrition pamphlet, "The Road to Wellville." From the very beginning, cereal advertisements have promised or implied good health.

When selecting a breakfast cereal we'd recommend the following guidelines:

- Select whole grain varieties: whole wheat, whole kernel corn, oatmeal, buckwheat, brown rice.

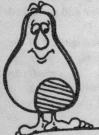

❋ CEREAL GLOSSARY

- **Whole Grain:** An entire cereal kernel which is ground, rolled, or cracked

- **Germ:** The seed or innermost part of a cereal kernel, rich in nutrients

- **Endosperm:** Surrounds germ and is rich in starch

- **Bran:** Outer layer which encases germ and endosperm, rich in fiber

- **Refined:** Bran or the germ or both have been removed

- **Enriched:** Restore some important nutrients (the three B vitamins and iron) that have been removed in refining

- **Fortified:** Adding one or more nutrients to a cereal that was either not present at all or that was not present in large amounts; vitamin D fortification of cereal is common

- Select cereals made from more than one grain; the grains complement each other and enhance the overall nutritional quality of the cereal, for example, Cheerios are made from oat and wheat flour.

- Select a cereal with less than 20 percent sugar.

- Vitamin- and mineral-supplemented cereals are expensive and of questionable nutritional value.

In a survey of 600 New York City school children Cheerios, Special K, and Wheaties were selected as favorite choices. You might try these low-sugar, "kid-tested" selections at breakfast. In the hot-cereal category, Maypo and Instant Quaker Oatmeal (regular flavor) were rated best in relative nutritional quality by an independent testing agency.

For additional information read through the remaining questions on cereal in this section.

Q *How can you tell which cereals have fiber?*

As awareness of the benefits of fiber in the diet has increased, cereal makers have begun to use the terms *fiber* and *bran* as marketing gimmicks. Over a dozen cereals contain the word *bran* in the title or mention *fiber* on the label.

Fiber is the indigestible part of plants. Good sources are whole grains, legumes (peas and beans), fruits, and vegetables. Children often eat limited quantities of dried peas and beans, fruits, and vegetables, but they readily eat cereal. Whole grain cereal or cereal with added bran would provide an excellent daily source of fiber and trace minerals. The laxative effect of fiber, especially wheat bran, can help to keep a child's bowel movements regular. Whole grain cereals like shredded wheat, oatmeal, Cheerios, Wheaties, All-Bran, Ralston, and Grape-Nuts are high in fiber. Refined cereals, made from the endosperm part of the grain, are high in starch and low in fiber—Cream of Wheat, Fruity Pebbles, Rice Krispies, Farina.

Other cereals that are whole grain or contain bran are:

Frosted Mini-Wheats	Quaker 100% Natural
Raisin Bran	Total
40% Bran Flakes	Maypo
Golden Grahams	Grape-Nuts Flakes
Wheatena	Crispy Wheats 'n Raisins
Nutri-Grain	Buc Wheats
Bran Buds	Cracklin' Bran
Pep	Graham Crackos
Most	

Read labels carefully. Look for the following terms: whole wheat, graham flour, whole kernel corn, rye, barley, buckwheat, rolled oats, and bran. Cereals, listing as their first ingredient wheat flour, degermed cornmeal, and milled rice are low in fiber.

Q *Should I let my little girl put sugar on her cereal in the morning?*

Presweetened cereals are more expensive than unsweetened varieties. If your daughter wants sugared cereal, we'd recommend adding the sugar at the table and not buying it in the box. One level teaspoon of sugar added to 1 ounce of Cheerios raises the percentage of sugar from 3 percent to 15 percent. This is still far below the amount of sugar in presweetened cereals.

One of the things we did with our children to discourage the use of too much added sugar was to leave a demitasse spoon in the sugar bowl. One spoonful of sugar per bowl was allowed but by using this small spoon the children were adding only ¼ to ½ teaspoon a serving. Cereals containing more than 10 percent sugar were tagged *sugared* and no extra sugar was added at the table.

Try adding fresh or dried fruit or a few drops of pancake syrup to hot cereal for added sweetness.

Q *My child begs me to buy highly sweetened cereal. Should I?*

The organization Action for Children's Television (ACT) has aggressively lobbied against deceptive cereal advertisements. These ads entice children with games of chance, premium purchases, and free gifts inside cereal boxes. Even the most resistant parent often gives in under this constant assault. To add insult to injury, it seems that the more highly sugared the cereal the more aggressively it is marketed.

We are not steadfastly opposed to some sugar in the diet. We believe an occasional serving of a sweetened cereal will not sabotage the health of a normal child. A breakfast featuring a presweetened cereal plus milk is better than no breakfast at all. Ideally, we'd like to see children eating a whole grain, unsweetened cereal. But more realistic is the hurried family breakfast or the argument in the supermarket featuring ". . . you never buy any cereal I like!"

Here are a few suggestions on how we've handled the issue of presweetened cereals with our own children. First, don't be afraid to counter deceptive advertising with the truth. Explain that prizes are put in sweetened cereals so that children will force their parents to buy them. Explain that a lot of sugar causes tooth decay and diets high in sugar are not healthy. Don't underestimate your child's ability to be an astute consumer. Karen, before she entered kindergarten, was frequently heard muttering at the television, "Why don't you put that toy in one of the *good* cereals!'' Second, be willing to compromise. Any forbidden food becomes more desirable. Buy a small box of the presweetened cereal. Explain that you feel it has so much sugar that it is really candy packed in a cereal box. Then dole it out as candy—as a snack, occasionally, and in small amounts. If the child insists on eating it as his breakfast cereal use it as a garnish to a more nutritious selection—a bowl of Wheaties topped with a handful of Lucky Charms. Third, explain that many cereals you buy, those with less than 20 percent sugar, are sweetened, but not with as much sugar as those that resemble candy. The chart Sugar Content of Some Cereals, page 58, will give you many good selections. See also the questions, ''Should I let my little girl put sugar on her cereal?'' and ''How can I tell if a cereal is presweetened?'' in this chapter.

Q *How can I tell if a cereal is presweetened?*

That isn't always easy. Most presweetened cereals announce their sugar content on the box with phrases like, *sugar coated, sugar frosted, ready-sweetened,* or *honey coated.* Apple Jacks, Cocoa Krispies, Lucky Charms, and Fruity Pebbles all have at least 40 percent sugar. Golden Grahams, Raisins, Rice and Rye, and Bran Buds are pushing fiber in their ads, yet they all contain at least 25 percent sugar.

When the word *sugar* appears on a food label it means only cane or beet sugar. Other sugary sweeteners are often added to cereals—corn syrup, honey, dextrose, molasses, brown sugar, invert sugar, maltose, and lactose. Ingredients are listed on the label in decreasing order of amount present. If sugar or a sweetener is first or second on the list, it's likely to be a highly presweetened cereal. For additional information see the chart Sugar Content of Some Cereals, page 58, and the next question, ''How much sugar is there in corn flakes?''

Q *How much sugar is there in corn flakes?*

The chart Sugar Content of Some Cereals, page 58, tells you that Kellogg's Corn Flakes have 5 percent sugar. Most cereal labels do not state the percentage of sugar in their product, however, they voluntarily list the grams of sugar and starch. With this information, you can determine the approximate amount of sugar in one serving of a cereal without milk.

Following is an example label of an unsweetened breakfast cereal.

Carbohydrate information	1 oz
Starch and related carbohydrates	19 g
Sucrose and other sugars	3 g
Total carbohydrates	22 g

One gram is equal to about ¼ teaspoon of sugar. The unsweetened cereal above has 3 grams of sugar or about ¾ teaspoon of sugar per serving (1 ounce dry cereal = ¾ to 1 cup of cereal, which is an average serving).

If the cereal were a presweetened type a sample label would look like this:

Carbohydrate information	1 oz
Starch and related carbohydrates	10 g
Sucrose and other sugars	16 g
Total carbohydrates	26 g

If 1 gram equals ¼ teaspoon of sugar, this presweetened cereal has 16 grams of sugar, or 4 teaspoons of sugar per serving.

The chart Sugar Content of Some Cereals lists the percentage of sugar in many common cereals. These products, however, appear and disappear quickly from the supermarket shelves. Knowing how to figure out how much sugar there is in a serving from the carbohydrate information on the label will help you to make good cereal choices. We'd recommend buying those cereals with 20 percent sugar or less. This would equal about 1½ teaspoons of sugar or less per serving if you did not add additional sugar at the table. This would also represent 6 grams of sugar or less on the carbohydrate information label.

Sugar Content of Some Cereals

Product	Total sugar, %
Sugar Smacks (K)	56
Apple Jacks (K)	53
Froot Loops (K)	48
Raisin Bran (GF)	48
Sugar Corn Pops (K)	46
Super Sugar Crisp (GF)	46
Cocoa Krispies (K)	46
Frankenberry (GM)	44
Cocoa Krispies (K)	43
Cocoa Pebbles (GF)	43
Fruity Pebbles (GF)	43
Lucky Charms (GM)	42
Cap'n Crunch (QO)	40
Count Chocula (GM)	40
Frosted Rice (K)	39
Raisin Bran (K)	39
Sugar Frosted Flakes (K)	39
Alpha Bits (GF)	38
Honey Comb (GF)	37
Frosted Rice (K)	37
Trix (GM)	36
Graham Crackos (K)	35
Cocoa Puffs (GM)	33
Honey Nut Cheerios (GM)	33
Honey and Nut Corn Flakes (K)	32

Sugar Content of Some Cereals

Product	Total sugar, %
Country Morning (K)	31
Instant Quaker Oatmeal, maple and brown sugar (QO)	31
Golden Grahams (GM)	30
Cracklin' Bran (K)	29
C. W. Post, Raisin (GF)	29
C. W. Post (GF)	29
Nature Valley Granola (Fruit and Nut) (GM)	29
Raisin, Rice and Rye (K)	28
Frosted Mini Wheats (K)	25
Bran Buds (K)	25
Vita Crunch (OM)	24
Familia (S)	23
Quaker 100% Natural, Brown sugar & honey (QO)	22
Most (K)	21
Life, Cinnamon (QO)	21
100% Bran (N)	21
All-Bran (K)	18
40% Bran Flakes (K)	18
Pep (K)	18
Life (QO)	16
Team (N)	14
40% Bran (GF)	13
Grape-Nuts Flakes (GF)	13
Buc Wheats (GM)	12
Maypo 30-Second Oatmeal (SM)	11
Rice Krispies (K)	11
Maltex (SM)	11
Special K (K)	10
Product 19 (K)	10
Total (GM)	8

Sugar Content of Some Cereals

Product	Total sugar, %
Wheaties (GM)	8
Grape-Nuts (GF)	7
Corn Flakes (K)	5
Post Toasties (GF)	5
Kix (GM)	5
Cream of Wheat (N)	
Instant	5
Regular	5
Rice Chex (RP)	4
Corn Chex (RP)	4
Wheat Chex (RP)	4
Wheatena (SM)	4
Instant Quaker Oatmeal, regular (QO)	3
Farina (P)	3
Instant Ralston (RP)	3
Quick Quaker Oats (QO)	3
Old Fashioned Quaker Oats (QO)	3
Cheerios (GM)	3
Quick Grits (QO)	1
Shredded Wheat (N)	1
Nutri-Grain (K)	1
Puffed Wheat (QO)	0.5
Puffed Rice (QO)	0

Note: Letters in parentheses following product name indicate manufacturers: General Foods (GF), General Mills (GM), Kellogg (K), Nabisco (N), Organic Milling (OM), Pillsbury (P), Quaker Oats (QO), Ralston Purina (RP), Somalon (S), Standard Milling (SM).

Q   *Should I buy a vitamin- and mineral-fortified cereal for my children?*

In 1956, Kellogg added vitamin D to Corn Flakes and sales increased. Corn Flakes are still fortified with vitamin D today. In 1968, General Foods fortified Sugar Crisps with one-third of the daily requirement for certain vitamins to boost sagging sales. The new fortified cereal was called Super Sugar Crisp and sales rose. The concept of a cereal as a vitamin pill began to catch on in the early seventies.

Today many cereals are promoted as highly fortified—Total, Product 19, Most. Cereal ads claim one cereal has seven vitamins, another one eight and the next one, nine plus iron. These advertisements create a false impression of nutritional adequacy since the nutritional benefits of fortification are questionable. The mere addition of a vitamin or mineral to a food does not insure that the nutrient will be used by the body. Many factors affect how the body absorbs and uses nutrients, including the presence of other nutrients. In addition, "supplement" cereals are more expensive than those that are less highly fortified.

Q   *Are granola cereals better for children than regular dry cereals?*

Crunchy Granola originated in California in the 1960s. Most granola cereals are higher in protein and made from natural products. Granola cereals found in the supermarket are pre-sweetened, often containing 20 to 30 percent sugar. Remember, sugar, brown sugar, honey, and molasses are all "natural" so they do not take away from the preservative-free marketing appeal of granola.

In Part III, Kid-Tested Recipes, beginning on page 227, is a recipe for a variation of the original Crunchy Granola. Children will enjoy making this cereal themselves.

MILK

Q   *My preschooler refuses to drink milk. What should
I do?*

Most young children like milk. You might try simple tricks
to encourage your child to drink it. Serve very cold milk.
Some children like it with an ice cube. Others like it warm.
Use a very small glass, juice-size, so the amount is not over-
whelming. Don't offer milk as the child's only drink choice.
Offer juice at meals occasionally and save milk as a breakfast
and snack beverage. If these suggestions fail, try the milk
alternatives listed below.

A child four to six years old should be drinking at least 2
cups of milk a day or its equivalent in food. When food substitutes are made for milk, you are giving the child foods that
have the same approximate calcium value as milk. Calcium is
a major mineral found in bones and teeth. Children need a
steady supply of this important mineral to insure proper
growth. In addition to calcium, milk provides protein, two B
vitamins (thiamin and riboflavin), and vitamins A and D, all
of which are needed for good health. For more information
see the chart Know Your Dairy Products, page 63.

Instead of milk try

½ cup yogurt	= ½ cup milk
¼ cup evaporated milk + ¼ cup water	= ½ cup milk
1 ounce natural or processed cheese	= ¾ cup milk
½ cup cottage cheese	= ¼ cup milk
2 tablespoons cream cheese	= 1 tablespoon milk
½ cup ice cream	= ¼ cup milk
½ cup pudding	= ½ cup milk
½ cup custard	= ½ cup milk

Q *Is it all right for my child to eat his cereal without milk?*

Dry cereal can be a good snack choice that children enjoy. Some children prefer their breakfast cereal dry with a glass of milk on the side. That's fine.

Remember, though, that the nutritional value of any cereal is enhanced by the simultaneous drinking of milk, whether in the same bowl or served side by side at the same meal. Milk supplements the cereal's plant protein and rounds out the combination by contributing additional vitamins and minerals, most notably calcium.

Hot cereals made with water or very little milk will provide fewer nutrients than a bowl of cold cereal eaten with more milk. You might try cooking the hot cereal in milk or sprinkling a tablespoon of nonfat dry milk over each portion. Even the "instant" hot cereals can be reconstituted with hot milk instead of hot water.

Know Your Dairy Products

Whole milk • Fresh cow's milk with a fat content not less than 3¼% milk fat; most whole milk is approximately 4% milk fat.

Pasteurized milk • Milk that has been heat-treated to kill harmful bacteria.

Homogenized milk • Milk that has been mechanically treated to reduce the size of the fat globules so that the fat will not separate to form a cream layer at the top of the milk.

Fortified milk • Milk containing added amounts of those nutrients already found in milk; vitamins A and D and protein solids may be added.

2% Milk • Fresh milk which has had its fat content reduced to 2% milk fat.

Skim milk • Fresh milk which has had its fat content reduced; ordinary skim milk has a fat content of 0.5–1%; protein-fortified skim milk has additional milk protein added to it.

Nonfat dry milk • Made of fresh whole milk from which the water and fat have been removed, resulting in a fine textured powder.

Evaporated milk • Homogenized whole milk from which half of the water was removed, fortified with vitamin D and canned.

Sweetened condensed milk • Whole milk which has had 60% of the water removed and sugar added (40–45% of the condensed milk); used primarily in desserts.

Acidophilus milk • Pasteurized, low-fat milk cultured with bacteria (*Lactobacillus acidophilus*), which converts milk sugar, lactose, to lactic acid.

Lact-Aid cultured milk • Fresh milk treated with lactase enzyme which converts 90% of the milk sugar, lactose, to lactic acid; used by those with lactose intolerance.

Buttermilk • Originally the fluid left after butter churning; today most buttermilk is made from skim milk cultured with bacteria (*Streptococcus lactis*).

Sour cream • Pasteurized, homogenized cream cultured with bacteria (*Streptococcus lactis*), resulting in a gel; contains at least 18% milkfat.

Yogurt • A fermented milk product made with varying milk fat levels (0.5%–3.25%); often mixed with other ingredients like dry milk solids, cream, sugar, vegetable gums, flavorings, and fruit preserves.

Butter • Made from cream, containing 80–82% butterfat.

Natural cheese • Made by coagulating milk and separating the curd (solid part) from the whey (watery part). Classified as to moisture content: soft (cottage cheese), semisoft (Muenster), hard (cheddar), and very hard (Parmesan).

Processed cheese • Natural cheese is melted, pasteurized, and mixed with an emulsifier to produce a cheese that has a uniform texture and flavor; often many additional ingredients and or additives are included: with added milk, whey, or oil, processed cheese can be changed to cheese food or cheese spread.

Q   *Is it true that milk sold in plastic containers has lost all its vitamins?*

No, that's not true. The major nutrients that milk contributes to a child's diet are calcium and protein. Neither of these are affected by the milk container material. What you probably are referring to are commercials and ads that suggest that milk packed in cardboard containers has more vitamins than milk packed in clear plastic containers.

Unfortunately many marketing wars are waged on television and in the newspaper. If we believed every ad we heard or read, we'd all live in spotlessly clean homes, where we effortlessly prepared nutritionally superior, attractive meals for agreeable well-mannered children. What a dream! Let's examine more closely the milk container war and then you can decide for yourself whether to buy milk in a plastic bottle or cardboard container the next time you go marketing.

Research studies have shown that when milk is exposed to light and heat there is a change in the flavor and a decrease in the amount of certain nutrients. The neighborhood milkman once provided his customers a metal, insulated "milkbox" that protected the quality of his product between the time he delivered it and the time his customers woke up. Today most of us buy milk at the supermarket. This milk may be affected by fluorescent light in the dairy case, particularly if the milk sits in that case for long periods of time. Clear plastic containers allow light to penetrate the milk and destroy a small portion of the vitamins. Cardboard containers provide better protection, especially if they are printed with dark colored ink on the display panels and spout area. One must also consider how long milk remains in the dairy case exposed to fluorescent lighting. Many supermarkets report restocking display cases as often as every three hours, especially on busy shopping days. Short exposure shows very little if any nutrient loss. The storage dairy case in the supermarket stock room and your home refrigerator are lit with incandescent light which does not affect milk quality.

If this issue is a concern to you, we can make a few recommendations. In vertical dairy cases, milk on the sides near the front is sold more quickly than that in the center or rear. In reach-in dairy cases rows 2 and 3 are taken quicker than row 1 or back rows. Whether in plastic or paperboard containers, milk from these sections has had the least light exposure. At home, store milk away from the refrigerator door so that it is not bathed in light each time the door opens. Serve at the table only the amount that will be used, do not leave a gallon or half gallon in the morning sunlight during the breakfast meal.

VITAMINS AND MINERALS

Q *Does a four-year-old still need to take a daily vitamin?*

There is no harm in giving your four-year-old a daily vitamin supplement. Forty-seven percent of all children aged three to five in the United States take vitamins. If you give one, we'd recommend a vitamin supplement with iron, as the incidence of anemia is high among three- to five-year-olds. (See the question, "How can I tell if my five-year-old is anemic?" in this chapter.) In addition we'd recommend using a supplement formulated for children under age four. The vitamin/mineral doses are lower in this variety but sufficient to supplement reasonable food choices.

The term *supplement* is the key. Vitamins and minerals given in pill form should supplement those nutrients found in food, not substitute for them. Daily nutrient supplements are an insurance plan you may wish to give to your child. They are not a guarantee of good health or adequate nutrition. We've often recommended parents give supplements every other day. This insures that "little extra" in case the child does not eat as well as you'd like but does not set up a pattern of relying on a pill to provide what isn't eaten in food. (For more information see the question, "Which are the best vitamins for my children to take?" in this chapter.)

Q Can you explain the label on my child's vitamin supplement?

All vitamin labels are set up the same and contain a good deal of valuable information. A sample label is shown on page 68.

1. Recommended dosage. Too many vitamins can be dangerous. Don't give extra when the child isn't feeling well or the weather is threatening.

2. The U.S. Recommended Daily Allowance (U.S. RDA) is the most commonly used labeling guideline recommended by the Food and Drug Administration (FDA). The U.S. RDA represents estimated amounts of nutrients needed every day by healthy people.

3. International Unit (IU) is a form of measurement used for vitamins.

4. Some vitamins and minerals are measured in milligrams (mg) and micrograms (mcg). A milligram equals one-thousandth of a gram; a microgram equals one-millionth of a gram; there are 28 grams in an ounce.

5. Names of some essential B vitamins that are normally included in multivitamin supplements.

6. All medications should be kept safely away from children to prevent accidental overdose.

7. Date by which the supplement should be used. Using vitamins after their expiration date is not dangerous. Your child, however, may not be getting much benefit from them because they have reduced potency. A rule of thumb is that if

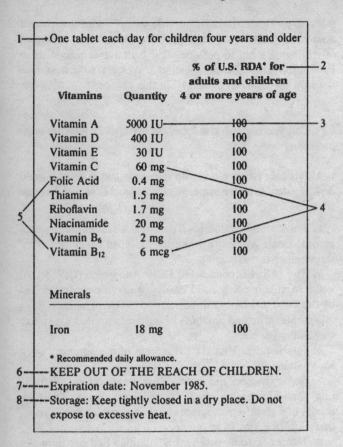

1 → One tablet each day for children four years and older

		% of U.S. RDA* for — 2 adults and children
Vitamins	Quantity	4 or more years of age
Vitamin A	5000 IU	100 — 3
Vitamin D	400 IU	100
Vitamin E	30 IU	100
Vitamin C	60 mg	100
Folic Acid	0.4 mg	100
Thiamin	1.5 mg	100
Riboflavin	1.7 mg	100
Niacinamide	20 mg	100
Vitamin B$_6$	2 mg	100
Vitamin B$_{12}$	6 mcg	100

Minerals

| Iron | 18 mg | 100 |

* Recommended daily allowance.

6 - - - KEEP OUT OF THE REACH OF CHILDREN.

7 - - - Expiration date: November 1985.

8 - - - Storage: Keep tightly closed in a dry place. Do not expose to excessive heat.

there is any change in color, taste, smell, or appearance you should discard them.

8. Vitamins should be stored in their original container, in a cool, dry place. The kitchen and bathroom are not the best places as the heat and humidity in these rooms hastens deterioration. A shelf in the linen closet or the top of the dresser is a better storage spot.

Q *Which are the best vitamins for my children to take?*

Many parents feel that as long as they give their child a daily vitamin supplement, that will make up for poor eating. Hardly! Vitamin/mineral pills are a *supplement* to food, not a *substitute* for it. We consider children's vitamin/mineral pills like an insurance plan or safety net—a guarantee that all bases are covered just in case your child doesn't eat as well as you'd like.

How do you select the right insurance plan for your child? The best place to start is by carefully reading the labels on the supplements you are considering. Before you can do this, you need to be an informed reader. On pages 67–68 we dissected a vitamin label for you. Now let's go one step further and help you compare the nutrients your child needs against what's offered in the supplement you are considering.

On the label you'll find a list of nutrients, the amount of each provided, and the percent of the U.S. RDA (U.S. Recommended Daily Allowance) each amount represents. For example, 2,500 I.U. of vitamin A equals 100 percent of the U.S. RDA for the vitamin.

The U.S. RDA is a nutrition-labeling tool. It gives a single amount for each nutrient. In most cases this amount is the highest value of the nutrient needed for any age or sex group. Many of the values reflect the needs of growing teenage boys. For young children, the U.S. RDA may be higher than their actual nutrient needs.

The RDA, Recommended Dietary Allowances, is a more precise guideline of nutrient needs. This standard is revised every five years and divides nutrient needs according to age and sex categories. Because of the many categories, the RDA is too cumbersome to use on a nutrition label.

Let's take a closer look at the U.S. RDA used on vitamin labels and the more precise RDA which recommends levels of daily nutrients needed by healthy children of different ages.

	U.S. RDA (nutrition-labeling tool)		RDA nutrient needs of healthy children		
	Children under 4	Children 4 years or older and adults	Ages 1–3	Ages 4–6	Ages 7–10
Vitamin A	2500 IU	5000 IU	2000 IU	2500 IU	3000 IU
Vitamin C	40 mg	60 mg	45 mg	45 mg	45 mg
Thiamin	0.7 mg	1.5 mg	0.7 mg	0.9 mg	1.2 mg
Riboflavin	0.8 mg	1.7 mg	0.8 mg	1.0 mg	1.4 mg
Niacin	9 mg	20 mg	9 mg	11 mg	16 mg
Calcium	800 mg	1000 mg	800 mg	800 mg	800 mg
Iron	10 mg	18 mg	15 mg	10 mg	10 mg
Vitamin D	400 IU	400 IU	400 IU	400 IU	400 IU
Vitamin E	10 IU	30 IU	5 IU	6 IU	7 IU
Vitamin B_6	0.7 mg	2.0 mg	0.9 mg	1.3 mg	1.6 mg
Folic Acid	0.2 mg	0.4 mg	0.1 mg	0.2 mg	0.3 mg
Vitamin B_{12}	3 mcg	6 mcg	2.0 mcg	2.5 mcg	3.0 mcg
Phosphorus	800 mg	1000 mg	800 mg	800 mg	800 mg
Iodine	70 mcg	150 mcg	70 mcg	90 mcg	120 mcg
Magnesium	200 mg	400 mg	150 mg	200 mg	250 mg
Zinc	8 mg	15 mg	10 mg	10 mg	10 mg
Copper	1 mg	2 mg	1.0–1.5 mg	1.5–2.0 mg	2.0–2.5 mg
Biotin	0.15 mg	0.3 mg	0.065 mg	0.085 mg	0.12 mg
Pantothenic acid	5 mg	10 mg	3 mg	3–4 mg	4–5 mg

You can plainly see that the nutrient amounts of the U.S. RDA for children over age four are higher, in most cases, than the RDA for preschool children. To see this clearly, compare the amounts in the second column with the recommendation in the fourth column. In every instance, except for vitamin D, the U.S. RDA is higher than the RDA recommendation for children four to six. Extra vitamins and minerals are unnecessary for healthy children and in some cases may be dangerous. Don't be fooled by ads for "high-potency" vitamins. Remember, your child is eating these same vitamins and minerals in foods. A supplement that supplies 50 to 100 percent of the RDA is more than enough for a healthy child.

Q *Is there any tonic or vitamin that will increase appetite?*

Through the years many foods and nutrients have been used as tonics, for a pick-me-up or to improve appetite. Arsenic tonics, rhubarb, cod liver oil, and thiamin have been tried. A severely malnourished child will have loss of appetite among other symptoms. In that case, appetite will return when the child receives vitamin/mineral supplements along with adequate food.

In the well-nourished child additional vitamins or minerals, whether given as a pill or a liquid, will not stimulate appetite. There are many reasons why a child's appetite is small — illness, stress, excitement, and slowed growth rate at this age. For more information see the Trouble Spots section in this chapter, beginning on page 38.

Q *How do I choose which vitamin supplement to buy for my children?*

That's not always easy to do. Television ads lead us to believe *all* children must take vitamins to be healthy. In some cases the ad implies that healthy children should be getting "extra C" or "more of the essential nutrients."

To decide which vitamin supplement to buy, we suggest closing your mind to the attractive packaging and the entertaining ads and considering only three factors: the list of ingredients, the form they are in, and the price.

The list of ingredients: In the preceding question we explained the difference between the U.S. RDA and the RDA. You now understand that the U.S. RDA is a labeling tool and not an accurate measurement of children's individual needs. The RDA is a more precise guide to the nutrient needs of healthy children. To help you compare a children's supplement against the RDA look at the chart Pick the Best Supplement on pages 74–77. We have compared popular children's supplements against the RDA. We've left a place for you to compare the supplement you are considering if it's not on the list. Pick a nutrient supplement that offers a wide variety of vitamins and minerals and does not offer a dose higher than 100 percent of the RDA. If the supplement you wish to use exceeds 100 percent of the RDA per dose, we'd recommend giving the supplement every other day, rather than daily.

The form of the supplement: Does your child prefer to drink his vitamins, chew them, or swallow them? This preference should be your guide to which form to purchase. One thing we'd like you to be aware of—some varieties of children's supplements are formulated with extra vitamin C. There is no conclusive proof that extra vitamin C daily makes a child healthier or free from colds. There is some evidence, however, that extra vitamin C given to children in chewable tablets may cause damage to their teeth. The pH of these chewable, vitamin C–containing tablets is acidic, similar to stomach acid, causing erosion of the tooth surface. Dental researchers advise that vitamin C supplements should not be given in a chewable form.

Price: Once you've decided on form and determined that the supplement provides a wide variety of nutrients, remember that the cheaper the cost per dose the better the buy. Divide the total retail price for the container by the number of doses supplied. For example, Centrum, Jr. costs $4.49 for a bottle of 60 tablets. One tablet is recommended daily; therefore, a daily dose would cost approximately 7 cents. Local, generic, or store brands are often less expensive, not because they are inferior to brand name supplements but because the price doesn't have to cover the cost of national advertising. The least expensive supplement is the best buy.

Q   *How can I tell if my five-year-old is anemic?*

Preschool children are more likely to be anemic than school-age children since many of the foods they eat are low in iron. When iron stores are low, the body cannot make enough hemoglobin to build new red blood cells. Since hemoglobin is bright red, the skin of a child who is anemic may become noticeably pale. Iron-deficient blood cells are small and these undersized cells can't carry enough oxygen from the lungs to the tissues. The entire body feels the effect. An anemic child may be tired, listless, irritable, and not feeling well. Many complain of headaches or stomach aches.

Children with low iron stores have shown behavioral changes such as hyperactivity, lessened attention span, and increased restlessness. Some researchers have even linked anemia to a reduced IQ. Behavioral changes, however, return to normal when iron levels are restored.

A curious side effect of anemia in some children is ice eating. Sometimes trays of ice are eaten every day. Eating non-food items is called *pica*. Ice eating stops almost immediately once iron supplementation is given.

Your doctor can tell if your child is anemic with a simple blood test. Most pediatricians have this done regularly as part

(Text continues page 78.)

PICK THE BEST SUPPLEMENT, CHILDREN AGES 4–6

Nutrient	RDA Children 4–6	Poly-Vi-Sol Chewable Vitamins	E.T. Children's Chewable Vitamins with Iron	Centrum, Jr. Vitamin/ Mineral Formula + Iron	Flintstones Children's Chewable Vitamins with Extra C	Shaklee* Vita-lea Chewables	Your Choice
Recommended daily dose		1 tablet	1 tablet	1 tablet	1 tablet	2 tablets	
Vitamin A	2500 IU	2500 IU	5000 IU	5000 IU	2500 IU	2500 IU	—
Vitamin D	400 IU	400 IU	400 IU	400 IU	400 IU	200 IU	—
Vitamin E	6 IU	15 IU	30 IU	15 IU	15 IU	15 IU	—
Vitamin C	45 mg	60 mg	60 mg	60 mg	250 mg	45 mg	—
Folic Acid	0.2 mg	0.3 mg	0.4 mg	0.4 mg	0.3 mg	0.2 mg	—
Thiamin (B_1)	0.9 mg	1.05 mg	1.5 mg	1.5 mg	1.05 mg	1.05 mg	—
Riboflavin (B_2)	1.0 mg	1.2 mg	1.7 mg	1.7 mg	1.20 mg	1.2 mg	—
Niacin	11 mg	13.5 mg	20 mg	20 mg	13.50 mg	10 mg	—
Vitamin B_6	1.3 mg	1.05 mg	2 mg	2 mg	1.05 mg	1.0 mg	—

Vitamin B$_{12}$	2.5 mcg	4.5 mcg	6 mcg	6 mcg	4.5 mcg	4.5 mcg
Biotin	0.085 mg	—	—	0.45 mcg	—	0.01 mg
Pantothenic acid	3–4 mg	—	—	10 mg	—	5 mg
Iron	10 mg	—	18 mg	18 mg	—	10 mg
Calcium	800 mg	—	—	—	—	160 mg
Phosphorus	800 mg	—	—	—	—	125 mg
Iodine	90 mcg	—	—	150 mcg	—	75 mcg
Magnesium	200 mg	—	—	25 mg	—	8 mg
Zinc	10 mg	—	—	10 mg	—	1 mg
Copper	1.5–2.0 mg	—	—	2 mg	—	1 mg
Molybdenum	0.06–0.15 mg	—	—	0.02 mg	—	—
Chromium	0.03–0.12 mg	—	—	0.02 mg	—	—
Manganese	1.5–2.0 mg	—	—	1 mg	—	—
Potassium	1525–4575 mg	—	—	—	—	100 mg

* Shaklee Chewables also contain 0.2 mg inositol.

PICK THE BEST SUPPLEMENT, CHILDREN AGES 7–10

Nutrient	RDA Children 7–10	Poly-Vi-Sol Chewable Vitamins	B.T. Children's Chewable Vitamins with Iron	Centrum, Jr. Vitamin/ Mineral Formula + Iron	Flintstones Children's Chewable Vitamins with Extra C	Shaklee* Vita-lea Chewables	Your Choice
Recommended daily dose		1 tablet	1 tablet	1 tablet	1 tablet	2 tablets	
Vitamin A	3000 IU	2500 IU	5000 IU	5000 IU	2500 IU	2500 IU	——
Vitamin D	400 IU	400 IU	400 IU	400 IU	400 IU	200 IU	——
Vitamin E	7 IU	15 IU	30 IU	15 IU	15 IU	15 IU.	——
Vitamin C	45 mg	60 mg	60 mg	60 mg	250 mg	45 mg	——
Folic Acid	0.03 mg	0.3 mg	0.4 mg	0.4 mg	.03 mg	0.2 mg	——
Thiamin (B₁)	1.2 mg	1.05 mg	1.5 mg	1.5 mg	1.05 mg	1.05 mg	——
Riboflavin (B₂)	1.4 mg	1.2 mg	1.7 mg	1.7 mg	1.20 mg	1.2 mg	——
Niacin	16 mg	13.5 mg	20 mg	20 mg	13.50 mg	10 mg	——
Vitamin B₆	1.6 mg	1.05 mg	2 mg	2 mg	1.05 mg	1.0 mg	——

Vitamin B₁₂	3.0 mcg	4.5 mcg	6 mcg	6 mcg	4.5 mcg	4.5 mcg	—
Biotin	0.12 mg	—	—	.045 mcg	—	0.01 mg	—
Pantothenic acid	4–5 mg	—	—	10 mg	—	5 mg	—
Iron	10 mg	—	18 mg	18 mg	—	10 mg	—
Calcium	800 mg	—	—	—	—	160 mg	—
Phosphorus	800 mg	—	—	—	—	125 mg	—
Iodine	120 mcg	—	—	150 mcg	—	75 mcg	—
Magnesium	250 mg	—	—	25 mg	—	8 mg	—
Zinc	10 mg	—	—	10 mg	—	1 mg	—
Copper	2.0–2.5 mg	—	—	2 mg	—	1 mg	—
Molybdenum	0.1–0.3 mg	—	—	0.02 mg	—	—	—
Chromium	0.05–0.2 mg	—	—	0.02 mg	—	—	—
Manganese	2.0–3.0 mg	—	—	1 mg	—	—	—
Potassium	1525–4575 mg	—	—	—	—	100 mg	—

* Shaklee Chewables also contain 0.2 mg inositol.

of your child's overall health care. If the child is anemic, your doctor will recommend an iron supplement.

If your child is placed on a supplement, give it as prescribed and store it safely. Too much iron can be harmful. After aspirin, the second most common cause of accidental poisoning among small children is taking iron supplements or vitamins with iron. As few as six to twelve tablets have been a fatal dose for a child.

See the chart Food Sources of Iron for more information and the question, "What about iron . . ." in Chapter 4.

Sources of Iron

Very good:	Good:
Liver	Egg
Beef	Avocado
Beans	Blueberries
Chili con carne	Chicken
Prune juice	Turkey
	Prunes
	Split peas
	Dry breakfast cereals
	Fortified hot cereals
	Whole wheat bread
	Green leafy vegetables

WORKING MOTHERS

Q *As a working mother, I try hard to fix a good evening meal but get discouraged when my 4½-year-old doesn't eat. What should I do?*

We are working mothers and the one thing all working mothers need to learn to do is *relax*. All the evidence clearly shows that children of working mothers, who are well cared for in the mother's absence, grow up fine. Yet we constantly worry. Food is a particular concern since the mother does not see what the child eats all day and gives the evening meal more importance. In a day-care or family-care setting, your child is probably eating a good, varied selection of foods. If he gets a hot lunch and afternoon snack, a large evening meal may not be appealing. Check with your sitter, center, or school to see what your child is eating during the day.

Here are a few facts about working mothers that you should know:

- Middle-income working mothers with young children have been suggested as the most receptive audience for nutrition education.

- Some research has found that employed mothers spend more time preparing food from scratch and home-based mothers use more convenience foods.

- The three most important factors that determine the food choices of working mothers are health, nutrition, and socialization of children.

Relax and keep up the good work.

CAUTIONS!

Q *My four-year-old occasionally nibbles the leaves of my houseplants. Is this dangerous?*

Most definitely! After medicines, plants are the leading cause of poisoning in children under age five. Most plant poisonings result in nausea, vomiting, cramps, and diarrhea but some plants are so poisonous that the consequences could be fatal. For example, when an oleander branch is used as a barbecue skewer enough of its potent digitalislike toxin can be transferred to the food to kill a small child. Dieffenbachia, "dumbcane," a popular houseplant, contains calcium oxalate which can burn the mouth, tongue, and throat, resulting in swelling that could obstruct breathing.

Children mimic your behavior. If you nibble on plants in the yard or park they will also. Poisonous moonseed berries closely resemble wild grapes. Autumn crocus has been confused with wild onion. Hemlock, which grows freely along the roadside, is commonly called "fool's parsley" or "false parsley." Its feathery leaves have been mistakenly eaten as parsley, its roots mistaken for wild carrots, and its dark seeds for anise. All parts are poisonous. The water hemlock, a close relative, has poisoned children blowing on pea shooters and whistles made from its hollow stem. Storing flower bulbs in the kitchen can result in an ingredient mix-up. In one case, daffodil bulbs were used as shallots in chicken stew, resulting in a very sick family.

Following is a list of some common poisonous plants and flowers. They need not be removed from the house or garden but children should be taught not to nibble their berries or leaves. If you ever suspect that your child has eaten a poisonous plant, call the nearest poison control center and your physician. If possible, get a sample of the plant for identification and attempt to determine how much was eaten. In most cases, the National Poison Center Network recommends vomiting be induced with syrup of ipecac. Proper medical care is always necessary in any case of suspected plant poisoning.

Poisonous Common Plants

Please don't eat the. . . .

Daffodils	Hens and chicken
Buttercups	Lupine
Bleeding heart	May apple
Caladium	Hemlock
Lantana	Water hemlock
Lily of the valley	Foxglove
Privet	Autumn crocus
Sweet pea	Jimson weed (thornapple, stinkweed)
Evergreen yew	Chinese evergreen
Oleander	Narcissus
Azalea	Jonquil
Mountain laurel	Rhododendron
Dieffenbachia	Philodendron
Delphinium	Amaryllis

Three

Food and the School-Age Child (Ages 7 to 10)

"Why is there so much anxiety over the young child's eating, when in adult life eating is one of the most enjoyable activities?"

—*Your Child's Food, 1934*
Miriam E. Lowenberg

Most recent evidence indicates that consumer awareness of food and nutrition is increasing. Whether this new awareness will filter down to children and result in good food choices and healthy eating habits is still an open question. Between ages 7 and 10, children start to separate from the family and become more independent. They begin making decisions that relate to food and food choices. With the influence of friends, the enticement of fast foods, and the hard sell of television and radio commercials, the school-age child needs sound information so he can make healthy food selections. Will he trade his sandwich at lunch for candy, eat green beans in the cafeteria at noon, or buy a soda on the way home from school? There will be many times when doing what everyone else is doing seems like more fun than doing what Mom and Dad have taught. In elementary school, children test values, reject some, and modify or incorporate others into their own sense of self. This move toward independence is one of the first steps in maturing.

During this same period, the growth pattern changes. The school-age child gains weight faster than height. Along with this weight gain, body proportions begin to change—fat tissue accumulates, muscles develop, bones thicken, some internal organs grow rapidly, the lung cage broadens and deepens, and the shoulders and hips grow wider. Pound for pound these growing children need more nutrients than adults, since they are getting ready for their final growth spurt during adolescence.

DAILY NEEDS

Q *Exactly what nutrients should I give my child each day?*

Children need a good variety of nutrients each day to support growth and development and supply the energy for their active lives. The chart Daily Food Guide for the School-Age Child will show you kinds of food your child should be eating daily.

Daily Food Guide For the School-Age Child

A school age child needs daily:

Milk

  2 cups
  1 serving = 1 cup

Use whole milk, evaporated milk (reconstituted with water), skim milk, nonfat dry milk, buttermilk, cheese, yogurt.

Meat, Fish, Poultry, and Protein-Rich Foods

  2 servings
  1 serving = 2 ounces *

Eggs, cheese, dried peas or beans, tofu, peanut, and other nut butters may be substituted for a serving of meat, fish, or poultry.

Vegetables and Fruits

  4 or more servings
  1 serving of vegetable = 1/3 cup
  1 serving of fruit   = 1 medium fresh fruit
                          = 1/3 cup cooked or canned fruit

1 serving of a vitamin C–rich food (orange, grapefruit, melon, strawberries, broccoli, tomatoes, and coleslaw).
1 serving of a vitamin A–rich food, dark green or deep yellow-orange in color (spinach, sweet potato, carrot, apricot, and mango).
2 or more servings of other fruits and vegetables (including potatoes).

Bread, Cereal, Rice, Pasta

  4 servings
  1 serving = 1 slice of bread
             = 1/2 cup cooked cereal, pasta, or rice
             = 1/2 cup dry cereal

Use only whole grain and enriched products.

* See page 85 for portion sizes of 2 ounces of protein.

Q *How big is the actual serving size for 2 ounces of protein?*

A 2-ounce portion of protein gives your child about 14 grams of protein. A school-age child needs approximately 34 to 46 grams of protein each day. Each of the following equals a 2-ounce serving and 14 grams of protein:

> 1 hamburger (3 inches diameter × ½ inch thick)
> 2 meatballs (1 inch diameter)
> 2 slices meat, chicken, turkey (2 inches × 2 inches × ¼ inch thick)
> 2 cubes of stew meat (1 inch square)
> 2 cubes cheese (1 inch square)
> 2 slices cheese
> 2 slices luncheon meat
> 1 frankfurter
> ½ cup cottage cheese
> 2 medium eggs or 1 large egg
> 4 tablespoons peanut butter
> 1 cup dried peas or beans
> 6 ounces tofu (soybean curd)
> 6 tablespoons peanuts

Q *Is it necessary to eat vegetables for good health?*

The per capita consumption of fresh vegetables climbed from 105 to 110 pounds in 1982. That is a 30-year high which is the continuation of a trend that started in the mid seventies. We would venture to guess that most of these gains were made from adults rather than children.

Vegetables contribute many valuable nutrients to the diet. Luckily, however, fruits can serve as an alternative nutrient source which children enjoy. If your child will eat fruits, allow him to substitute a fruit when a less favorite vegetable is served. Raw vegetables, like carrots, broccoli, celery, and peppers are more likely to be chosen than a cooked choice. Remember salads are vegetables too. Serve raw vegetables with a dip for dinner once in awhile or reserve a portion for your child before cooking. Our children enjoyed stir-fried vegetables because of their crisp texture and because it was a dish they could "cook."

A school-age child should be eating four or more servings a day of vegetables and/or fruits. Juice or fruit for breakfast, a fruit for lunch, and a fruit and potato at dinner easily meets this requirement. As children grow older, most become more sophisticated eaters and they begin trying vegetables. Adults who refuse to eat vegetables were often forced to eat them as children. Don't make an issue of not eating vegetables, just provide reasonable substitutes and time will correct the problem.

HUNGER AND LEARNING

Q *My fifth grader is very active. Somedays he doesn't eat till supper. Is this harmful?*

Children's bodies need a regular source of energy (calories) which comes from the food they eat. When your son goes all day without food, his body has limited energy available. It will be difficult to eat all the calories he needs in the evening so he may be short on calories and nutrients. In areas of the world where growing children are chronically undernourished these children never reach their full growth potential.

Studies have also shown that children who fast for brief periods, even as short as three hours, made more errors on tests. The ability to concentrate and learn is directly related to how well nourished the body is. Brain function can be affected by subtle changes in nutritional status.

A child like yours should take the time to eat, not only for nourishment but to learn to relax and reduce stress. We've made many suggestions for quick meals and snacks. See A Dozen Breakfasts, page 131, the question, "What are some good snacks to give my daughter after school?" on page 90, the section on school lunch in this chapter, and the following question, "Are hunger and learning related?"

Q Are hunger and learning related?

It has been estimated that as many as 25 percent of all school children come to school without having eaten breakfast; many others do not have lunch. These children are frequently hungry. *Hunger* results when not enough food is eaten to meet immediate energy needs. Hunger is easily relieved with food and does not cause long-range growth problems unless coupled with malnutrition (prolonged intake of inadequate amounts and/or kinds of food). For most school children in this country, hunger is a more common problem than undernutrition. Nevertheless, hunger can have long-term effects on learning and behavior development.

The hungry child will often do poorly in school. Hunger dulls the child's interest in and ability to learn from new experiences. Skipping breakfast or lunch causes apathy, a shortened attention span, and disruptions in class. Teachers and classmates react negatively to this, isolating the child even further. Being hungry may lead to a decreased sense of self-worth and social isolation. The hungry child fails to learn because of environmental and psychological reasons rather than for biological or neurological reasons. The net result, however, is the same—the hungry child will not achieve his full potential.

When hungry children were offered midmorning milk the teachers reported a decrease in "nervousness." When milk plus food was given there were dramatic improvements in fatigue, excitability, attention span, and sociability. In a school breakfast study of boys, work rate and work output were increased during the period the boys ate breakfast at school. Many studies have suggested that school feeding programs have decreased student sleepiness and apathy while improving attitudes, awareness, and school performance.

Hungry children can't learn, therefore we need to help children understand why it is important to take the time to eat meals and snacks during the school day.

Q Is there any harm in a child skipping breakfast in the morning?

Having read this far in the book, you must have noticed that we are breakfast advocates. Children who skip breakfast tend to be overweight, they exercise less, and they eat more salt than children who eat breakfast regularly. Breakfast eaters also have significantly lower blood pressures. Results of several studies suggest that eating breakfast benefits the child emotionally and enhances his ability to work on school tasks.

Breakfast should offer a child approximately one-fourth of his energy and nutrient needs for the day. This translates to between 325 to 500 calories, depending on the child's size and age. Below are some typical breakfast patterns:

½ cup whole milk	80 calories	
½ cup dry cereal	110 calories	
6 ounces orange juice	60 calories	
1 slice bread	70 calories	
1 teaspoon jelly	17 calories	
Total	337 calories	
1 cup whole milk	160 calories	
½ cup dry cereal	110 calories	
6 ounces orange juice	60 calories	

1 slice bread	70 calories
1 pat butter	45 calories
1 teaspoon jelly	17 calories
Total	462 calories

2 fried eggs	216 calories
1 cup whole milk	160 calories
6 ounces orange juice	60 calories
1 slice bread	70 calories
1 pat butter	45 calories
Total	551 calories

An occasional skipped breakfast will not hurt a healthy child. Also keep in mind that breakfast food need not be the traditional milk and cereal. Your child might enjoy munching on a cold chicken leg on the way to the bus stop. It is not important what the child eats for breakfast but that he eats. For some novel breakfast ideas see the question, "My daughter hurries out to school each morning missing breakfast. . . ." in Chapter 4.

SNACKING

Q *Why does my nine-year-old eat very little at dinner and then beg for snacks all night long?*

At this age it is typical for a child to get intensely involved in a game, television, or a project. They often become so engrossed in an activity that mealtimes become an intrusion. This is the child who must be called repeatedly before he comes to dinner. Once at the table he eats a small amount hurriedly, claims to be full, and begs to be excused. If allowed to leave the table, he'll be back looking for food before the dishes are washed. If forced to sit while the rest of the family eats he'll fidget and spill something, annoy siblings, and become a general disturbance until banished.

He wants after-dinner snacks because he is still hungry and needs more food to make up for the unfinished meal. This isn't an easy phase to deal with, but, in fact, it's only a phase and it will pass. You might try a compromise. Tell your child you expect him to come to the table promptly when called. You'll allow him to be excused, however, when he is "full" and he can come back at the end of the meal for dessert. He should be asked if he'd like more dinner, first, when he returns for dessert. Many times these children eat in shifts—a first helping, 15 minutes later a second helping, and finally dessert.

There is nothing wrong with allowing this child a substantial bedtime snack—cereal and milk, cheese and crackers, peanut butter on toast—since he is not overeating but just finally found the time to eat.

Q *What are some good snacks to give my daughter after school?*

School-age children love after-school snacks. Many enter the front door, drop their bookbag, and go to the refrigerator before they say hello or take off their coats. We used to watch in amazement the amount of food Steven ate when he got home from school. Almost 40 percent of all children have an after-school snack.

Many of us grew up with the idea that snacking spoils the appetite and isn't consistent with good nutrition because it interferes with meals. Scientific research doesn't support this. Children who snack often have a leaner build and are better nourished than their nonsnacking counterparts. The suggestion is that snackers eat when they are hungry rather than when the clock designates a mealtime. Snack foods add to the total daily nutrient intake contributing 20 percent of the calories, 12 percent of the protein, and between 10 and 20 percent of many other needed nutrients.

Grade-school children list bakery products (mainly cookies), soft drinks, candy, fruit, milk, salty snacks, milk desserts, and bread as their favorite after-school snacks.

The following are some snack ideas you might offer your daughter:

Open-face toasted cheese sandwich
English muffin pizza
Waffle and a scoop of ice cream
Cereal and milk
Bowl of soup and crackers
Hot chocolate and cinnamon toast
Apple Graham Cracker pudding*
O.J. Tapioca*

See the sections on snacking in Chapters 1, 2, and 4 for more ideas.

* See Part III, Kid-Tested Recipes.

Q *Is peanut butter a good food?*

Most children enjoy peanut butter. Some seem to live on it, never tiring of a daily peanut butter sandwich. You really needn't worry, since this is one food you can let your child eat each day. Two tablespoons of peanut butter can substitute for one ounce of meat, fish, or poultry.

Peanut butter is regulated by federal standards of identity and must contain 90 percent peanuts. Additional ingredients may include salt, sugar, stabilizers, and oil. Artificial flavors, artificial sweeteners, chemical preservatives, and added vitamins and coloring are forbidden by law.

You might also want to try those peanut butters made only from peanuts, either prepackaged or ground to order. These products are more expensive than commercial peanut butter but many consider them worth the extra cost.

To add some variety to the traditional peanut butter sandwich try mixing any type of peanut butter with one of the following:

peanut butter + mashed banana
              + raisins
              + honey
              + cottage cheese
              + pureed canned fruit
              + cooked dried fruit
              + applesauce
              + ricotta cheese
              + shredded cheddar cheese
              + shredded coconut
              + prune butter
              + apple butter
              + poppyseed pastry filling

Q *Are seeds a good snack?*

Sunflower, pumpkin, and squash seeds are good sources of fiber, protein, calcium, and many other nutrients. For a child who is watching his weight, buy seeds in the hull. Peeling off the outer hull to get at the edible seed slows down the act of eating. We'd recommend the unsalted varieties.

At Halloween, your child might enjoy making his own toasted pumpkin seeds. Scoop out the pumpkin seeds and wash in a colander under running water. Spread on paper towels to dry. Lightly oil a shallow pan and spread out pumpkin seeds. Bake at 250°F for one hour, stirring occasionally. Store in a closed container.

Q *Should I buy juices packaged in cardboard boxes?*

The "paper bottle" was introduced in 1982. It was designed as a replacement for the single serving can or bottle. Drinks packed in the paperboard container do not require refrigeration, making them versatile as a snack-on-the-go or for lunch. Drinks packed in foil-lined pouches are also available.

Both of these products are safe to use. We would recommend buying only those that are unsweetened juices—orange, orange-pineapple, grape, apple, grapefruit, and fruit punch. Many of these pouch or boxed products are "drinks"—a sweetened beverage with a very small percentage of fruit juice. *Capri Sun* advertises its pouch drinks as "made with 10 percent fruit juice and nothing artificial." Their ad is correct, the *Capri Sun* pouch drinks are basically sugar, water, and a little fruit juice. These products are long on calories and short on nutrients.

The flavor of these juices is enhanced when chilled. Freeze them overnight and they will defrost slowly in a lunch box, helping to keep the entire lunch chilled until it's time to eat at noon.

SUGAR

Q *Which foods are high in sugar?*

Before we answer that, let's talk a little about sugar. What is it? What does it do to our children's health?

A lot of people think Winnie the Pooh was on to something when he was searching for the honey pot. In actuality, sugar is sugar, whether it comes from the sugarcane, sugar beet, or the beehive. The human digestive tract responds to all of these sugars in the same way. No one sugar can be singled out as "good" or "bad" for your child. The chart Sugar, Sugar Everywhere, on page 95, will explain the many types of sugar we eat. All sugars listed in this chart are similar in calorie content.

White sugar has been characterized as a "killer" responsible for everything from hyperactivity, to obesity, heart disease, and diabetes. There have even been suggestions that eating sugar could contribute to delinquency in children. We think that most of these reports are not grounded in scientific fact and must be viewed with skepticism.

Sugar may be classified as an *empty calorie* food in that it contributes little else but calories. Even honey and brown sugar, which contain a few traces of nutrients, would have to be eaten in large amounts, over a cup a day, before they would make a substantial contribution to the diet. A cup of brown sugar contains 740 calories and a cup of honey contains 1,034 calories. Herein lies the problem. Sugar calories can substitute for more nutritious calories in the diet of a child: an orange drink rather than orange juice; iced cake rather than a slice of bread; a soda rather than milk. The development of a sweet tooth can lead to a habit of eating high-calorie, sweet foods which might contribute to obesity and tooth decay. Sugar calories burn off quickly, leaving a child feeling sluggish and hungry. Slower-burning calories from protein or fat will make the child feel fuller longer.

If a child eats a wide variety of foods an occasional sweet will do no harm. Sugar is a problem only when it is eaten in such large amounts that it substitutes for better foods or adds too many calories to the diet.

The issue of sugar in children's diets is very complex. We addressed the issue in many places. See Chapter 2 for more information on the sugar content of breakfast cereals; Chapter 6 for the role of sugar in tooth decay; Chapter 7 for information on artificial sweeteners; Chapter 8 for sugar's use as an energizer for athletes, and Chapter 9 for sugar and allergies. Also see the charts Sugar Content of Some Cereals, page 58, and Sugar in Snacks, page 97.

Sugar, Sugar Everywhere

Granulated sugar • White crystals refined from the sugarcane or sugar beets; all traces of molasses are removed.

Powdered sugar • Finely ground granulated sugar packed with a small amount of cornstarch to prevent caking; also called *confectioner's sugar*.

Raw sugar • The sugarcane is crushed and refined to the point where it is separated into blackstrap molasses and raw sugar crystals; raw sugar is illegal in the United States because it contains bacteria, insect fragments, and dirt.

Turbinado sugar • A cleaned and partially refined light brown coarse, crystal sugar; often called *sugar in the raw*.

Brown sugar • Granulated sugar moistened and colored with molasses-flavored sugar; also available in a pellet form.

Molasses • The thick liquid produced in the refining of sugar.

Blackstrap molasses • The final syrup extracted from the sugarcane during refining; strong-flavored and contains some minerals.

Corn syrup • Produced from the breakdown of cornstarch to form a thick, sweet liquid.

Honey • A liquid sugar made up of glucose and fructose, made by the honeybee from the nectar of flowering plants.

Maple syrup • Condensed and boiled sap of sugar maple trees.

Pancake syrup • A mixture of all or some of the following: artificial flavor and color, corn syrup, maple syrup, and honey.

Sorghum • A cane-like grass yielding sugar; syrup may be prepared from the juice of sorghum.

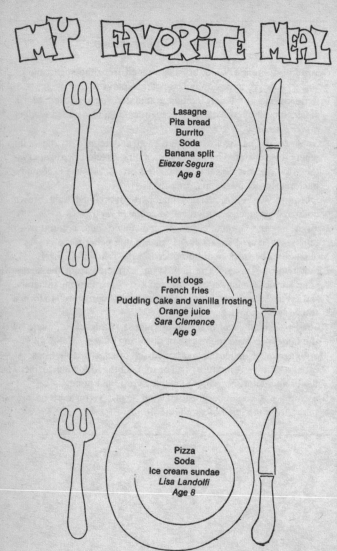

MY FAVORITE MEAL

Lasagne
Pita bread
Burrito
Soda
Banana split
Eliezer Segura
Age 8

Hot dogs
French fries
Pudding Cake and vanilla frosting
Orange juice
Sara Clemence
Age 9

Pizza
Soda
Ice cream sundae
Lisa Landolfi
Age 8

Sugar in Snacks

Food	Serving size	Teaspoons per serving of sugar
Lifesavers	1	1/3
Cool-Whip	1/4 cup	4/5
Fruit Roll-Ups	1	1 7/8
Cracker Jacks	1/2 box	3
Canned pears in heavy syrup	1/2 cup	3
Hershey Milk Chocolate	1 ounce	3
Jelly beans	10	3 3/4
Strawberry jam	1 tablespoon	4
Lollipop	1 small	4
Pop Tart (sugar/cinnamon)	1 tart	4
Brownie	1 square	4
Tang	4 ounces	4
Hunt's Vanilla Snackpack	1 pudding cup	4 1/2
Jell-O	1/2 cup	5
Fig Newtons	1 cookie	5
Milky Way	1 regular-size bar	5 3/4
Kool-Aid	8 ounces	6
Apple cider	8 ounces	6
Frozen pudding pop	1	6 1/2
Raisins	1/4 cup	8
Coca-Cola	12 ounces	9

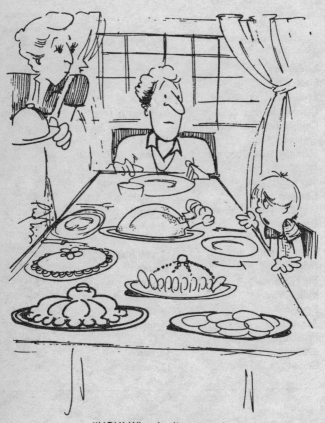

"UGH! Why don't you ever
make anything I like!"

SCHOOL LUNCHES

Q *Are school lunches nutritious?*

Students who buy and eat lunch at school receive 31 to 43 percent of their recommended daily nutrients. Children who bring lunch from home or buy an alternate to school lunch get only 17 to 26 percent of their daily needs. Furthermore, school lunch is a bargain, costing less than a comparably nutritious meal brought from home.

Read through the remaining questions in this section for more information.

Q *Are there guidelines for what is served for school lunch?*

The National School Lunch Program began in 1946 in order to provide school children with a nutritious meal which meets one-third of their daily nutrient requirements. Many of you grew up eating Type A school lunches. The Type A lunch has grown up too and is now called the lunch meal pattern. The nutrition principles used to feed you as children have not changed dramatically. The school lunch served each day must consist of five items:

   2 ounces of a meat or a meat alternate
   ¾ cup total of fruit and/or vegetable (this serving *must* be provided by two foods, such as one fruit and one vegetable)
   1 serving of whole grain or enriched bread, pasta, rice, noodles, or other bread alternates
   8 ounces fluid milk

These sample school lunch menus would meet the five-component lunch as follows:

Food item	Sample menus		
Meat/meat alternate	Oven-fried chicken	Hamburger on bun	Pizza with cheese topping
Vegetable or fruit	Mashed potatoes Green beans	French fries Apple	Apple juice Salad
Bread/bread alternate	Roll	(Hamburger bun)	(Pizza crust)
Milk	Milk	Milk	Milk

In addition to the basic five components, modifications have been made in the lunch foods to control fat, sugar, and salt in the children's lunches. Salt and sugar packets are not allowed to appear on the lunch service line; canned vegetables are packed in a lowered salt brine; canned fruits are packed in light syrup rather than heavy syrup or replaced by fresh fruit; low-fat milk has replaced whole milk in many cafeterias or both are offered, and sugary or fatty snacks and desserts are eliminated or at least limited. Today, when the children get peanuts, they are *unsalted*!

For your school to continue to be a member of the National School Lunch Program and receive reimbursements, it must follow all these federally mandated regulations, and it does!

Remember: The basic purpose of school lunch is to serve our children a nutritious, attractive meal in a pleasant environment. The lunchroom provides a learning laboratory for the classroom, where nutrition concepts can be put into practice. We should encourage its use.

Q *I just got a notice from my child's school stating that the children will no longer have to eat their whole school lunch. Why?*

Your school district has probably just approved "offer versus serve" guidelines for the school lunch program. This option can only be adopted on the elementary and junior high school level by the approval of the local school board. The normal lunch meal pattern consists of five items. When "offer versus serve" is adopted, the children have the option of taking only three or four of the items offered. For example:

Traditional lunch pattern (no choice)	Offer versus served (student choice)	Traditional lunch pattern (no choice)	Offer versus served (student choice)
Pizza + cheese	Pizza + cheese	Oven-fried chicken	Oven-fried chicken
Apple juice	Apple juice	Green Beans	Peaches
Salad	Salad	Peaches	Roll
Milk		Roll	Milk
		Milk	

This regulation was instituted in 1982 to reduce food waste while maintaining the consumption of a variety of different and nutritious foods by students. When it was mandatory to take all items in the school lunch pattern, children simply threw out those they would not eat. Many argued that this system encouraged plate waste. With "offer versus serve" the children are taught to "take what you want and eat what you take." When an unfamiliar food is offered a "taste it" portion can be given and the child may come back and have more. Of the three items picked, each item must be a different lunch component. A child could not take three servings of french fries as lunch. The "offer versus serve" option recognizes that students have food preferences and trusts the student with the responsibility to choose those foods he intends to eat.

Q *Our school lunch menu resembles the food at McDonald's. Is this healthy for the children?*

In order to get children to eat school lunch it must compete with the fast food alternates. Remember, though, that as long as the school is a member of the National School Lunch Program it must meet all federal guidelines. (See the question in this chapter, "Are there guidelines for what is served for school lunch?")

Some schools are not members of the federal lunch program and some have opted to offer a la carte items in addition to the regular lunch. Here is where parental pressure counts. Find out what is being served and make your wishes heard. Many schools have stopped the sale of candy and soda. A school district in Massachusetts has allowed the McDonald's chain to open a lunch program in a vocational high school. The traditional McDonald's fare, however, was modified somewhat to comply with parental wishes.

Q *What are some good lunches I can make for my son to take to school?*

Many lunches are made each school morning but how many are actually eaten at noon? To minimize the chance of your child's lunch landing in the trash, consider these points:

1. A child is less apt to discard a lunch he makes himself.

2. Children should be allowed to help plan what goes in their lunch box.

3. Respect your child's concern about peer pressure. He doesn't want to feel different at the lunch table even if it is a food he normally loves.

4. Teach your child nutrition principles so he understands what foods make up a good lunch.

A nutritious lunch for a school-age child should include

8 ounces of milk
2 ounces of protein

1 fruit or vegetable
2 slices of bread or alternate

With a wide-mouth thermos, an insulated lunch bag and a few small, lidded plastic dishes, lunchtime can be full of surprises and good taste. See the chart A Dozen Interesting School Lunches, below.

A Dozen Interesting School Lunches

Yogurt
Walnuts and raisins
Oatmeal cookies
Cranapple juice

Cut-up fruit
Cottage cheese
Whole wheat crackers
Brownie
Chocolate milk

Chicken noodle soup
Whole wheat bread sticks
Cheese cubes
Carrot sticks
Fig Newtons
Milk

Chili con carne
Corn muffin
Bunch of grapes
Milk

Franks and beans
Tossed salad
Pound cake
Milk

Cold chicken leg
Cole slaw
Granola bar*
Milk

Pita Salad Sandwich*
Banana
Chocolate pudding*
Apple juice

Peanut butter and jelly on
    cinnamon/raisin bagel
Pear
Milk

Bologna and American cheese
    on rye
Macaroni salad
Hot chocolate

Raw vegetables and dip
Sesame crackers
Rice pudding
Grape juice

Stew	Hot cereal
Rye bread	Fresh fruit
Celery sticks	Banana bread
Milk	Orange juice

* Recipes in Part III, Kid-Tested Recipes.

Q *I spend time making tasty school lunches only to have my son announce he "traded" at lunchtime. How can I stop this?*

Don't. Trading school lunches broadens young food tastes. Eating with classmates may be a youngster's first experience "dining out." Eating away from the parent's watchful eye opens up an exciting world of foods and combinations of foods children would not go near, let alone taste, at home.

We remember Karen's delight when her friend Keiko taught her to eat sushi and cold rice with chopsticks. We can assure you, she'd never have considered eating raw fish if her mother had made it! We've heard tales of onion-and-rye bread sandwiches, pancake-jelly roll-ups, blintzes in a thermos, and cold pizza.

As a parent you can't help feeling secretly annoyed when you hear how well "so-and-so's" mother makes lunch. Relax, "so-and-so's" mother is probably just as tired of hearing about you!

Q *My fourth-grade daughter refuses to carry a lunch box because it's "babyish." What do I do?*

That's not unusual. About age nine, many young girls begin to assert how independent they are and how "grown-up" they can act. Lunch boxes are for "little kids." Many insulated bags are designed for adult lunches. Perhaps your daughter would like one of these. If not, look for a small plastic or canvas shopping bag. Remember to pack the food so that it will stay cool till lunch. See the question in this chapter, "My daughter loves tuna salad sandwiches but I'm afraid they'll spoil in her lunch box" for suggestions on how to do this.

If a thermos is "out," try a single-serving juice or buy milk at lunch. Many schools have milk and juice on sale in the lunchroom.

If your daughter wants a "brown bag" lunch buy those waxed brown bags you see at the supermarket designed especially as lunch bags. Bags you get from stores should not be used as lunch bags. These leftover bags have been shown to be unclean. Some were never intended to carry food and have traces of insect droppings and larvae that could contaminate the lunch.

Q   *My daughter loves tuna salad sandwiches but I'm afraid they'll spoil in her lunch box. Will they?*

No. Tuna salad is no more likely to spoil than any other food. You may mistakenly believe that foods containing mayonnaise spoil quickly. Mayonnaise is not the culprit. Its high acidity provides an excellent antibacterial barrier and, in fact, protects foods it is in contact with from spoilage. The real problem is the protein foods—chicken, eggs, tuna, meat, and fish. Their low acid content makes them ripe for bacterial growth in a warm environment. Make your daughter's tuna salad from cold ingredients. You can either make the tuna salad the night before or simply refrigerate the can overnight. Pack her lunch in an insulated bag. If it will be many hours till lunch, include a small picnic ice gel or make your own by freezing water in a tight-lidded plastic dish. Freezing paper-boxed or foil-pouched juice acts like an ice pack till lunch. A small, reusable, first-aid ice pack also makes a good "lunch box refrigerator." Remind your daughter not to store her lunch box on the classroom radiator; a cool coat closet is a much better place.

TELEVISION AND EATING

Q *Does television influence my child's food choices?*

It most certainly does. Television has been called the "first curriculum" and its influence cannot be underestimated when one realizes that 90 percent of all American three-year-olds can recognize Fred Flintstone.

The average child watches 25 hours of television a week, adding up to between 8,500 and 13,000 food and beverage commercials a year. There is little doubt that this advertising affects the food preferences of children and ultimately the food purchases made by parents. When food commercials were categorized during a sample week, almost 70 percent of the commercials were devoted to products high in fat, cholesterol, sugar, and salt. Only a fraction of advertising, 1 percent, promotes foods such as fruits, vegetables, or dairy products.

In addition to the advertising barrage, the subtle message on prime-time television, daily soap operas, and children's shows is "live for today." Television and cartoon characters pay little, if any, attention to their own health but suffer few ill effects. They lead unhealthy lifestyles, eat and drink to abandon, and rarely exercise. Yet, despite all this, they remain healthy, sober, safe from accidents, and slim at all ages. An analysis of one week's programs found fewer than 6 percent of the males and 2 percent of the females were obese, whereas in reality 25 to 45 percent of Americans struggle with this problem. Television characters eat, drink, or talk about food an average of nine times per hour but never gain an ounce!

Those networks that aired the largest number of comedy shows, which attract the biggest viewing audiences, had major characters who ate the greatest proportion of less nutritious foods.

Children need to understand the difference between make-believe television characters and real life. Further, they need to gain an understanding of how television advertising works so they can make sound consumer decisions in a marketplace containing a growing number of confusing choices.

See the next question for more information.

Q *How can I counteract the food ads my child sees on television?*

Food advertising literally surrounds us—on television and radio, in newspapers and magazines, on billboards, buses, and trains—and we can't ignore it. The purpose of advertising is to inform, educate, and ultimately sell a product. You must recognize, that in the eyes of a marketer, your child is part of a "target group."

Before you can combat food advertising on television, you'll need to teach your child the purpose of a commercial. Many young children don't recognize a difference between the sponsor and the program. A child views a total program, accepting the commercial as a part of the show. To help distinguish between the two, Action for Children's Television (ACT) was instrumental in ending the practice of using program hosts to promote products.

Help your child evaluate foods he sees on television: Don't be afraid to state your own opinions: highly sweetened cereals are not good breakfast choices; fruits make a better snack than candy; homemade dinners taste better than canned spaghetti. Explain that premiums are offered in cereals or through box-top promotions to increase sales. Explain advertising techniques. A snazzy racing car climbing backyard mountains on a television ad performs far differently from the one-inch model they'll find in the cereal box. Point out that "They want the car to look exciting so that children will ask for the cereal."

Don't be afraid to set some limits: In our homes there are certain products we just don't buy. Our children know this and don't ask for them. "Requesting behavior" (the marketing term for nagging) on the part of children is directly proportional to how often parents follow through with purchases. If you don't want your child to nag for certain foods, don't buy them. It works. Don't feel guilty about your vetoes. You control the food your child eats, not the television advertiser.

Listen to requests for new foods: If you have set good food standards your child will know this. Therefore, if he requests a television food, look at it together next time you shop for groceries. Read the label. If it meets your standards, try it at least once. Allow your child to have some input about what the family eats. You'll be surprised that your child may introduce you to many new and interesting foods that are nutritious as well.

Don't feel you are at the mercy of food ads that offend you: Write to the appropriate parties. The action of concerned parents and others has had an impact on children's television: advertising on children's shows has been cut by 40 percent; cereal commercials must show a complete breakfast, not just the cereal being advertised; and to discourage misuse or overuse, vitamins are no longer advertised on children's programs.

See the section on cereals in Chapter 2 for some additional helpful consumer information.

BAKE SALES

Q *Are there any good money-making ideas that can substitute for the traditional school cake sale?*

It is interesting how mothers complain about sugared cereals, candies, and cakes, and then turn around and volunteer to bake for a school cake sale. There are some recipes that are appropriate for bake sales—corn muffins, raisin whole wheat muffins, carrot cake, and oatmeal cookies, just to name a few.

But why not be adventurous and offer the children something new to try? A fruit sale is fun. Crisp autumn apples are delicious, oranges in the winter, and plastic bags of cherries in the spring. Declare one day a month "Popcorn Day." Sell small bags of freshly popped corn. Vary the seasonings for interest—garlic salt, pizza spice, grated cheese, even cinnamon-sugared popcorn for dessert.

Children also enjoy interesting snack foods. Try selling

- nuts and dried fruit
- cheese cubes and crackers
- large soft pretzels
- dry cereal, coconut, and nut mix

In one school the innovative chairman of the ways and means committee has a monthly "Snacks by the Ounce" sale. PTA volunteers set up a table filled with plastic containers full of nuts, peanuts, dry cereal, shredded coconut, raisins, dried fruit, small pretzels, popcorn, chocolate chips, and sunflower seeds. The children are given a small sandwich bag into which they scoop any snack mixture they wish. Their snack mix is weighed, on a small kitchen scale, and the children are charged by the ounce. Parents are happy to give their children money to purchase these healthy snacks and the school has an ongoing fund raiser that no one objects to.

Note: In some schools, sales begin before lunch, in which case children buy and eat before lunch. Plan the sales so they do not replace lunch.

EATING OUT

Q *We love to eat out but the children frequently waste what they order. What can we do?*

We both fondly remember the first time we took our children to a restaurant and no one spilled something in our lap and we didn't spend half the meal in the rest room. Eating out with young children often winds up as a challenge rather than a treat.

From a child's point of view, dining out is not always a wonderful event. It means long boring stretches between courses, unfamiliar foods, and scoldings to sit up, sit still, and stop pouring the salt all over the table. What is most discouraging is that children rarely eat much of what they've ordered and you've paid for.

Here are some ideas we've tried after many years of eating out with our children:

- *Pick restaurants where children are welcome and can be comfortable.* Diners, pancake houses, fast food chains, and family style restaurants are meant for families and used to children. Your choice can become more elegant as the children get older.

- *Ask for a children's menu.* Many places offer alternate choices, like hamburgers or grilled cheese, even when not listed. Do not hesitate to inquire.

- *Ask if children may share a meal.* One adult meal may serve two children nicely, particularly if they have different tastes. One may want the soup, the other salad, dividing the selections happily.

- *Ask if a la carte service is available.* A complete dinner, not eaten, is no bargain. It may be cheaper to buy only what the child wants and will eat. At one time, Karen's favorite restaurant served her an a la carte dinner of soup, a baked potato, and a dish of ice cream.

- *Never insist a child try a new food when eating out.* Children are far less inhibited than adults. They'll make a face, spit the food out, and proclaim how "awful" the lobster is.

- *Skip the parsley.* Never be afraid to ask for a naked hamburger—without garnish, lettuce, or tomato. The lettuce only winds up in the ashtray or balanced at the edge of your plate. Ask for vegetables, gravy, or salad on the side. That will spare you the chore of wiping runny coleslaw off fried chicken.

- *Hold the drinks.* Ask that the beverages be served with the meal, not before. The same goes for bread and butter. Let each child have a roll or split one between two children. Then ask the waiter to remove the bread-basket.

- *Plan to wait.* A pad and pencil or a hand-held video game can make waiting between courses much easier. Many family style restaurants provide place mats with puzzles or pictures to color.

WORKING PARENTS

Q *Our work schedule is such that we leave home too early to give the kids breakfast. Any suggestions?*

Today's family schedule makes it difficult for families to eat breakfast together at home. Fifty-eight percent of all mothers with school-age children work outside the home. As working mothers, we know how hectic mornings can be and we share your concern that a good breakfast is an essential part of starting the day. The key is, how do we get the time to make it and feed it to the kids, especially if we are dashing out the door when they are half awake.

We can offer some ideas. First, don't be afraid to make the children responsible for breakfast. Teaching children basic domestic skills makes them feel very responsible and is important if they must spend some time alone at home. Cold cereal and milk is a "help-yourself" breakfast which does not require the use of home appliances. Instant hot cereal can be prepared if you fill a child's thermos with boiling water before you leave. We especially like the type with a pour-spout lid which minimizes the chance of spills. Sandwiches for breakfast are also easy, "fix-yourself meals" or perhaps yogurt or cottage cheese and fruit.

Many communities have before-school programs at local YMCAs or YMHAs where children receive adult supervision and breakfast. Many schools serve breakfast as an extension of the National School Lunch Program. These meals are very inexpensive and offer the child a three-component breakfast each day: a juice or fruit, a milk, and a whole grain or enriched bread or cereal. Many schools offer additional a la carte items to enlarge the basic choices. Most children enjoy breakfast at school and eat more when in the company of friends.

Q *What suggestions can you offer a working mother to help provide good suppers?*

The traditional family—employed father, nonworking mother, and at least one child under 18 living at home—exists in only 15 percent of American households. The shift away from the traditional family structure has caused changes in eating styles—more meals away from home, less meal planning, fewer meals eaten together as a family, and a greater reliance on convenience foods.

We've both worked and managed families simultaneously and we know the panic that sets in around dinnertime. We've often wondered if working fathers worry if there is milk in the refrigerator while they are in a business meeting.

Regardless of whether you are a single mother or a married woman with a cooperating spouse, meal planning and preparation still seems to remain a woman's responsibility. Women seem to feel guilty if they don't cook and feed their families. Please realize that nutritious meals need not be gourmet fare. Toasted cheese sandwiches on whole wheat bread and waldorf (apples, walnuts, raisins) salad is a wholesome dinner choice. Convenience foods, well-chosen, can be very helpful when time is short. If you and your husband eat large business lunches and the children get a hot lunch at school, a small, simple dinner is a good choice.

Older children who get home first can be called upon to start dinner. Laura, Allen, and Steven often do this when mother is late. Younger children can help set the table, break up salad greens, peel carrots. Karen and Kristen at five and seven could produce terrific Italian bread pizza. The bread was cut in half lengthwise and the cheese pregrated. They totally prepared the pizza and made a salad with prewashed salad ingredients on the night they and their father got home first. Stir-fried vegetables and boneless chicken can be ready in minutes. Serve it over rice, and dinner is complete. Jo-Ann relies on her freezer a great deal, always cooking for two meals—making extra spaghetti sauce or two casseroles at once. She also freezes leftovers in small covered casseroles and on nights when there is no time to cook, reheats for the family a smorgasbord of past dinners. Crock pot cooking is very helpful to a working mother. Dinner is begun in the morning and is waiting, piping hot, when you get home. There are many excellent cookbooks to help you with ideas.

If all else fails—you've gotten home too late, and nothing has been planned for dinner—serve breakfast. It may sound like a crazy idea but it's not. Scrambled eggs, toast, and fruit is a quick and very nutritious meal. Or try French toast, waffles, or an omelet. During the week, most busy families don't have time for large breakfasts, yet they enjoy those foods. Why not offer some breakfast favorites for dinner?

PROBLEMS

Q *My eight-year-old son and I constantly fight over what he should eat. How can I stop this?*

Food choices can easily become a power struggle between a parent and child. We can assure you that your situation is not unique. What is needed is a new way of communicating about food. Then the child learns to make good food choices, eliminating the power struggle that ends with you screaming, "Eat it because it's good for you!" or "Eat it or else. . . ."

Below are some examples of food conversations that will illustrate this situation:

Mother: "Here's your cereal."
    Son: "I hate breakfast!"

Mother: "You have to eat something before you go to school."

Son: "No, I don't."

Mother: "Yes you do or you won't watch any television tonight."

Son: "I'm not eating that cereal!"

Mother: "You have to eat if you want to learn in school."

Son: "Who wants to learn anyway!"

This situation probably escalates into a full-fledged screaming match and even if the child does eat, both he and his mother are full of anger, resentment, and frustration that may color the rest of their day.

Good conversations with children are a skill that must be based on respect. The skill comes with repeated practice, resulting in good communication. The messages sent from parent to child must preserve both the parent's and child's self-respect. Statements of understanding must *precede* statements of advice or instruction.

The boy who refused breakfast was not communicating with his mother. Their conversation was two alternating monologues, one consisting of threats and instructions, the other of defiance and anger.

Let's look at a new approach to that same conversation:

Mother: "Here's your cereal."

Son: "I hate breakfast!"

Mother: "You hate to eat breakfast."

Son: "I hate cereal!"

Mother: "You hate to eat cereal for breakfast."

Son: "I hate to have to do all that chewing first thing in the morning."

Mother: "You'd rather eat something that doesn't make you chew so much."

Son: "Yeah, how about a bowl of soup."

The boy didn't hate breakfast, he simply did not like the choice presented. With the second conversation the mother let her end of the conversation mirror what she thought the child was saying or feeling. This technique is nonjudgmental and opens the door for further communication. It takes practice to become skillful at *hearing* what the child is actually saying but the result will be less confrontation over food.

Here is another example of a good conversation about food choices:

Mother: "Eat some green beans."
   Son: "No, I hate vegetables!"
Mother: "You hate green beans."
   Son: "Yes, they are mushy and have no taste."
Mother: "You don't like vegetables that are mushy."
   Son: "I like crunchy things like salad."

In this situation, which could have resulted in a power struggle over whether or not to eat vegetables, the mother's skillful mirroring of the boy's responses helped her find out that there were alternate choices he would have eaten. Perhaps in the future she could offer a salad or raw green beans.

With the help of a skillful dialogue, blanket declarations by children about food such as "I hate breakfast" or "I won't eat vegetables" can be turned into conversations that will point out alternate food choices that children will eat that are reasonable as well as nutritious.

Always remember that as long as your child eats a variety of foods his meal choices do not need to be the usual or traditional ones (like cereal for breakfast) and the combinations he chooses do not have to be the most typical (meat loaf, mashed potatoes, and plums are fine).

Q   *I've heard that some children have high blood pressure. Is this something I should be concerned about?*

All parents should be informed about the risks for hypertension, especially if there is a history of high blood pressure or heart disease in the family. Hypertension affects 2 to 4 percent of all children in grammar school. For this reason, children should have their blood pressure taken during routine medical visits as a simple screening measure. It is extremely unlikely that your child will have high blood pressure at this age. As he or she grows older, however, there is a one in six chance that hypertension will develop. This condition, which often shows no symptoms, is a major risk factor leading to heart attack, stroke, and kidney failure. For more information see the question, "Several members of the family have high blood pressure. . . ." in Chapter 4.

Four

Preteens
(Ages 11 to 13)

*"For school children the diet
should be varied and abundant,
constantly bearing in mind that this
is a period of great mental and physical growth."*

—*The Boston Cooking-School Cook Book,*
Fannie Farmer, 1896

The preteen years, ages 11 to 13, are a time of rapid growth for girls and many boys. By age 12, half the girls have reached the peak of their growth spurt and half of the boys have begun their spurt of intensive growth. The time of greatest growth is usually 11 to 13 for girls and 13 to 15 for boys. This growth is most obvious as you see them spurt up and become taller. We remember when Allen seemed to grow up and out of his jeans every few weeks. There is also organ and muscle development that may be less noticeable.

Nutrient needs are high. In fact girls 11 to 14 need more calories than at any other time in their lives. For boys the peak need is later, at ages 12 to 22. If these needs are not met, the growth spurt will be delayed or reduced. Yet studies show repeatedly that 13-year-olds have the poorest diets of any age group.

Anyone who is close to a preteen cannot help but notice that this is also a time of emotional highs and lows, as the child is learning how to "fit" his maturing body. Emotional instability, besides interfering with eating, causes greater loss of calcium, nitrogen (protein), and vitamins A and C from the body. You can plainly see the need for these and other nutrients.

Preteens become more independent, eating meals and snacks away from home. They often do not want guidance on how to make the best food choices and the choices they make are not based on the healthfulness or nutrient content of the food. Selections are more likely a result of peer pressure, enjoyment, sociability, status, advertising, or concern with appearance. Soft drinks are named as the favorite food.

It's often hard to convince preteens that their health, energy level, and appearance reflect what they eat. They do not relate food eaten to their present and future health. They think nutrition is boring and not really relevant. They are so overwhelmed with present needs that they show little concern for what may affect their future health.

Attempts to teach preteens about what to eat often fail because the approach, either too authoritarian or too childishly simplistic, does not appeal. It is far better to focus on the preteen's interest in being tall, slim, attractive, athletic, and also to take into account food preferences and the social implications of food. Nutrition education won't work when taught in a vacuum.

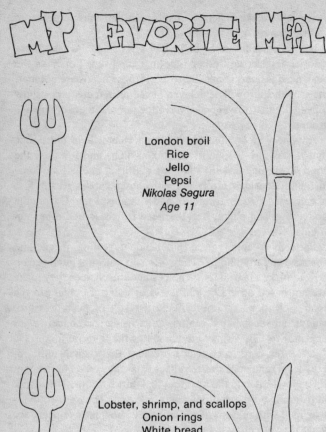

MY FAVORITE MEAL

London broil
Rice
Jello
Pepsi
Nikolas Segura
Age 11

Lobster, shrimp, and scallops
Onion rings
White bread
Hawaiian punch
Ice cream cake
Marc Jensen
Age 11

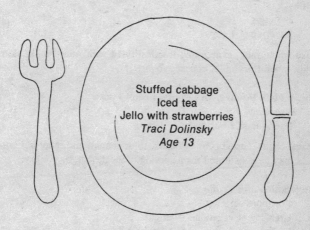

Stuffed cabbage
Iced tea
Jello with strawberries
Traci Dolinsky
Age 13

DAILY NEEDS

Q *How can I get my preteen more interested in good food choices?*

Preteens are experiencing rapid growth and change in their bodies and minds. They struggle to cope with these and at the same time gain acceptance from their peers. They know that attractive looks, a trim body, muscles (for males), and athletic ability will get them the approval and acceptance they seek. When they can be made to understand the role that food plays in achieving these desired characteristics and in making them feel good about themselves, better eating will follow.

Advice on what to eat would be readily accepted from rock stars, radio and television personalities, and athletes. Educa-

Daily Food Guide for the Preteen

A preteen needs daily:

Milk

    2–3 cups
    1 serving = 1 cup

Use whole milk, evaporated (reconstituted with water) milk, skim milk, nonfat dry milk, cheese, yogurt.

Meat, Fish, Poultry, and Protein-Rich Foods

    3 servings
    1 serving = 2 ounces*

Eggs, cheese, dried peas or beans, tofu, peanut, and other nut butters may be substituted for a serving of meat, fish, or poultry.

Vegetables and Fruits

    4 or more servings
    1 serving of vegetable = ½ cup
    1 serving of fruit   = 1 fresh fruit
                           = ½ cup cooked or canned fruit

1 serving of a vitamin C–rich food (orange, grapefruit, melon, strawberries, broccoli, tomatoes, and coleslaw).

1 serving of a vitamin A–rich food, dark green or deep yellow-orange in color (spinach, sweet potato, carrots, apricots, and mango).

2 or more servings of other fruits and vegetables (including potatoes).

Bread, Cereal, Rice, Pasta

    4 or more servings
    1 serving = 1 slice bread
                 = ½ cup cooked cereal, rice, or pasta
                 = ½ cup dry cereal

Use only whole grain and enriched products.

* See page 85 for portion sizes of 2 ounces of protein.

tors frequently point to the success of soft drink commercials that use heroes to deliver the message. Unfortunately, nutrition advice normally comes from teachers, parents, or health personnel who lack glamour. That is why the advice is likely to be rejected.

One good way to motivate preteens is to involve them, both boys and girls, in family food purchases and meal preparation. Why not have your preteen cook dinner one night a week? We remember one summer when Allen worked for a takeout caterer and prepared gourmet family dinners from what he had learned. They were delicious and included foods that the other children tried only because their big brother made them. Many schools offer popular courses in nutrition and cooking. Try to interest your child in one. Another ploy is to enlist help from the physical education teacher or coach. When they relate good eating with improved athletic performance preteens may take notice.

Parents should become involved in providing nutritious snacks to the participants of after-school and extracurricular activities. When the parents of Kristen's little league baseball team were asked to bring cold drinks to the games, the first drink brought was soda. After a discussion with the coach, he agreed that better choices should be provided. Juice, milk, fruitade, and flavored milk became standard refreshments. By the end of the winning season, the team was convinced that their drinks had a lot to do with their success.

NUTRIENT NEEDS

Q *Is there a special need for calcium during the preteen years?*

Yes, there is a time when increased amounts of calcium are needed, 1,200 mg daily, more than at any other time and as much as is needed during pregnancy and breast-feeding. This is because the bones are growing so rapidly. Adequate calcium is needed for healthy bones now and in the future. Research shows that a low intake of calcium during rapid growth periods reduces bone growth and may also make the person more susceptible to thin, weak bones (osteoporosis) later in life. That is why it is doubly important for your child to consume foods that are rich in calcium. Teenage boys drink large amounts of milk. It is their second favorite snack food. Teenage girls, however, drink far less than they need, often less than 2 cups a day.

Few foods are excellent calcium sources. Milk is an obvious choice, as 1 quart (4 cups) contains over 1,000 mg (1,000 mg = 1 g) but there are other good choices too. Preteen girls especially should be encouraged to eat calcium-rich foods each day because they are growing so rapidly now. See the charts Sources of Calcium, below, Instead of Milk Try . . . , page 62, and Know Your Dairy Products, page 63.

If your child gets a stomachache after drinking milk see the information on lactose intolerance in Chapter 9.

Sources of Calcium

Very good:	Good:
Milk	Tofu
American cheese	Ice cream
Swiss cheese	Mozzarella cheese
Cheddar cheese	Custard
Sardines	Salmon
Yogurt	
Collards	

Fair:
Cottage cheese
Broccoli
Spinach
Shrimp
Almonds

Q *What about iron? I have heard that many adolescent girls become anemic.*

Low iron intake is usually noted as the most serious deficiency in adolescence. The rapidly growing child is building blood and muscle that call for iron. Even though girls use less iron for growth than boys they have a further need for iron to replace the amount lost in menstruation. Girls who eat little food so that they can lose weight are at a greater disadvantage. The average balanced diet provides 6 milligrams of iron for each 1,000 calories, and poor diets may have less than that. The RDA for both boys and girls of 11 and over is 18 milligrams. This would be obtained on the average in 3,000 calories. Active boys may eat that much or more but if a girl is on a reducing diet eating less than 1,500 calories a day she will not be getting enough iron. That is why an iron supplement is often recommended for adolescent girls.

The most common form of anemia is caused by iron deficiency. Folic acid and vitamin B_{12} deficiencies are less often the cause. However, you don't have to be anemic to be low in iron. Low iron stores can cause weakness, irritability, depression, restlessness, reduced resistance to infection, and even anxiety. Some researchers believe that children who are iron-deficient have reduced ability to learn and have behavior problems.

When possible, it is better to meet iron needs through food because large doses of iron can be harmful. Iron-rich foods are liver, beef, turkey, pork, beans, prunes, and spinach. Iron is one of the nutrients added to enriched flour and cereals. You can increase the iron content of foods by cooking it in iron pans.

Only a small percentage of the iron in food is absorbed, so how much is absorbed is as important as the iron content. Until you absorb the nutrient it is really still outside your body even though it is in your digestive tract.

Absorption depends on several factors; one is the type of iron. All of the iron in grains and vegetables is called *nonheme* and it is poorly absorbed compared to *heme* iron. About 40 percent of the total iron in meat, fish, and poultry is *heme* iron; the remaining 60 percent is *nonheme*.

Absorption is affected in other ways as well. When iron is needed, the body will absorb more. Eating a vitamin C–rich food (orange, grapefruit, tomato, potato) or some meat, fish, or poultry at a meal will increase the amount of *nonheme* iron absorbed from all food at that meal. Adding a tomato to a hamburger meal quadruples iron absorption.

Drinking tea and coffee with a meal will reduce the quantity of iron absorbed and so will EDTA (ethylenediamenetetra-acetic acid), a food additive.

Q *Should I give my daughter an iron supplement?*

You have surely seen the commercials that stress the importance for an iron supplement for menstruating girls. It is truly difficult, if not impossible, for an adolescent girl to get all the iron she needs in her food. That is why it may be a good idea to give your daughter an iron supplement. Iron is available in liquid or tablet form.

Multivitamin preparations with iron usually contain 18 mg. Some iron supplements planned especially for females have 20 mg in each tablet. One tablet of either of these daily is sufficient. Your daughter should not take more unless recommended to do so by your doctor. High intakes of iron can be dangerous.

Iron supplements can be taken with food or between meals. There are advantages to both. Absorption is best when taken on an empty stomach. Some people develop stomachache, constipation, diarrhea, or nausea from the iron. These side effects are reduced when the preparations are taken with meals. Some tablets are available coated (enteric-coated) so that they do not irritate the stomach. Less iron is absorbed in this form.

Ferrous iron compounds are absorbed better than ferric compounds. Ferrous fumarate, ferrous sulfate, and ferrous gluconate are available and all are equally effective.

Q *Does nutrition affect the age of onset of menstruation?*

Yes, it appears to. The average age of menarche (first menstruation) in England around 1850 was 15½ to 16½. The average age of menarche in the United States is now less than 12½. This is two years earlier than at the turn of the century. That reduction in age is attributed to better nutrition. It might even be possible to relate it to a single nutrient.

Recently, two physicians (O. James Giannini and Andrew E. Staby) developed a theory that related the eating of citrus fruit to earlier onset of menstruation. They report that during the Renaissance, girls who lived in the south of Italy began menstruating at age 12, while those living north of the Alps had menarche at age 16; exercise, exposure to sunlight, and diet were similar except for citrus, which could not be shipped well over the mountains. Girls whose families moved north and no longer had citrus fruits available had delayed menstruation similar to their new neighbors.

The scientists also pointed out that the reduction in age of menarche in the United States was first noted in the 1920s. Self-squeezed orange juice was introduced here in 1916. Another large increase in use of orange juice occurred after World War II, and again it was accompanied by another decline in the age of menarche.

Q *What other nutrients are likely to be missing in my preteen's diet?*

Besides the minerals iron and calcium, the nutrients most likely to be in short supply are vitamin A and to a lesser degree vitamin C, thiamin, and riboflavin. The reason for these deficiencies is that kids eat highly processed foods, lots of fast food, and little fresh fruits and vegetables, whole grains, and milk. Skipping breakfast reduces the supply of some of these nutrients too. The chart on page 129, A Preteen's Missing Nutrient Menu, will show you how to help your child fill in these nutrient gaps. It is better to rely on food for this rather than a supplement. Supplements, if needed, should be additions to food, never a substitute for it. Two glasses of milk or the equivalent in cheese or yogurt, a serving of dark green or yellow vegetables, and some citrus fruit or juice will go far to make up the missing nutrients.

Q *My preteen children love to eat in fast food restaurants. Is this a good idea?*

People have been enjoying fast foods since the days of Pompeii. They are available, convenient, moderately priced, and taste good. Unfortunately many of the choices are very high in calories, fat, salt, and sugar, and low in fiber and some vitamins and minerals. More careful selections, like milk instead of a soft drink, a plain hamburger instead of one with all the trimmings, and a salad from the increasingly available salad bar (easy on the dressing) instead of fried potatoes can convert a fast food meal or snack into a more useful contribution to your child's daily food intake. It's also a good idea to round out a fast food meal by choosing fruits, vegetables, and other low-fat foods in meals and snacks during the rest of the day. Here are some suggestions on how to balance out your fast food meal. Let's use the Chinese restaurant menu approach—one selection from column A, one from column B—to fill in nutrient gaps.

A PRETEEN'S MISSING NUTRIENT MENU

Column A (foods with vitamin A)	Column B* (foods with calcium)	Column C (foods with vitamin C)	Column D (foods with iron)
Milk	Milk	Orange	Eggs
Eggs	Cheese	Grapefruit	Breads
Sweet potato	Tofu (soybean curd)	Strawberries	Cereals
Spinach		Cantaloupe	Turkey
Collards	Broccoli	Tangerine	Baked beans
Broccoli	Shrimp	Watermelon	Prunes
Squash	Sardines	Coleslaw	Apricots
Cantaloupe	Spinach	Potato	Avocado
Peach	Collards	Tomato	Chili
Apricot	Yogurt	Broccoli	Nuts
Carrots	Ice cream	Green pepper	Bologna
Mango	Custard	Papaya	Fried Chicken
Needed for healthy skin and eyes	Beans Needed for healthy bones and teeth	Needed for healthy gums and skin	Needed for healthy blood and muscles

* The dairy foods in this group also contribute needed riboflavin to the preteen's diet.

If you have eaten:
Hamburger + coleslaw
    add: 1 from Column A
        1 from Column B
Pizza + cola
    add: 1 from Column A
        1 from Column D
Hot dog + french fries
    add: 1 from Column A
        1 from Column B

Roast beef sandwich + vanilla shake
    add: 1 from Column A
        1 from Column C
Taco + fried onion rings
    add: 1 from Column A
        1 from Column B
        1 from Column C
Fried chicken + mashed potatoes
    add: 1 from Column A
        1 from Column B

BREAKFAST

Q *My daughter hurries out to school each morning missing breakfast. What can I do?*

We have all heard over and over about how important breakfast is, yet it is often hard to make time for this meal in the morning rush. Your preteen would rather spend the time combing her hair or dressing, and besides, she says, she's not hungry anyway (she's watching her weight) and the bus comes early.

Breakfast is truly an important meal. The body needs nourishment in the morning because it has not been fed for eight hours or more. Breakfast supplies nutrients that may be lacking in other meals, such as the vitamin C in orange juice. It also usually includes carbohydrate (sugar or starch) that can increase blood sugar so that slow reaction time is less likely. Students who skip breakfast take longer to make decisions, their work output is lower, and their muscles are not as steady.

In spite of all this, breakfast is the meal most likely to be skipped, and the likelihood of skipping it increases with age. If your daughter is passing up breakfast to lose weight she might be surprised to learn that obese adolescents are more likely to skip breakfast than kids whose weights are normal.

Don't think about breakfast only in terms of traditional foods like fruit, cereal, eggs, toast, or pancakes. Although these will make a good meal, you may be able to entice reluctant eaters with something a little more novel. Why not try some of the following. . . .

A DOZEN BREAKFASTS

Stand-ups	Time to eat	No hurry
Banana milk shakes	Scrambled eggs in	Pizza Scramble*
Apple and Granola Bar*	pita bread pockets	bagel
Orange juice and handful	English muffin and	Cheesy pancake
of nuts and raisins	melted cheese	roll-up*
Raisin bread and peanut	Yogurt and graham	melon
butter	crackers	Create a quiche*
	Cold chicken and	Meat loaf sandwich
	whole wheat toast	on rye toast
		orange sections

* Recipes start on page 231.

SNACKING

Q *My 13-year-old snacks all the time. I worry that he may not be getting all the nutrients he needs.*

Your son is in good company, studies show that 75 percent of all teens snack frequently. These snacking teens get up to one-fifth of all their calories this way. Although many usual snacks like chips and soft drinks may provide little except energy (calories), many snacks actually chosen by kids are nutritious. Here are the favorites of boys and girls given in order of preference:

Boys		Girls	
Soft drinks	Milk desserts	Soft drinks	Fruit
Milk	Salty snacks	Bakery	Milk
Bakery	Meat	products	Candy
products	Fruit	Milk desserts	Bread
Bread		Salty snacks	Meat

You can see many good snacks listed. There are others. Why not try . . .

- Whole wheat sesame bread sticks
- Cooked pudding with peanut butter*
- Yogurt sundae: try topping it with nuts, sunflower seeds, wheat germ, raisins, or fresh fruit
- Apple wedges spread with peanut butter or served with cheese slices
- Whole grain muffins
- Create a Crunch*

Relax, studies show that adolescents who eat more often than three times a day have better diets than those who eat less often. As a matter of fact, 12-year-old boys eat six or more times a day. Remember that kids tend to eat whatever is readily available, so keep a supply of nutritious snacks in your home.

Q *Is it all right for kids to eat a lot of salty chips?*

A study of school children aged 5 to 12 found that a large number of them ate no salted snacks during the week. The children who did eat salty snacks ate only a moderate amount and these occasional snacks did not affect the children's diets, which were adequate.

A study of teenagers aged 13 to 18 showed similar results. The average amount eaten by those who ate salty snacks was 3.1 ounces—two to four small packages a week. This amount had little effect on the average intake of nutrients each day. In fact, the teens who ate moderate amounts of salty snacks had

* Kid-Tested Recipes, page 227.

more nutritious diets than those who did not eat any. Preteens consider salty snacks a favorite food but it is not their top snack choice.

While nutritional intake may not be adversely affected by eating salty chips, there are reports that some adolescents are consuming alarmingly high intakes of salt. In fact a recent study of college students showed that they were eating more than the amount considered safe, even when excluding salt added from the saltshaker.

Q *What is junk food?*

We don't like to single out foods and label them as *junk* because foods really must be considered as a part of the total diet. Foods that are high in calories and low in nutrients, like soft drinks, dips, candy, and pastries, have been called *junk foods*. But if these foods are eaten in small amounts, occasionally as part of a well-rounded, varied diet, we'd rather that they be considered less desirable food choices. Eaten in this way, they will not sabotage an otherwise good diet.

Often those foods which are considered "fun foods" are low in nutritional value. We wouldn't want to label them as *junk,* as they add to the pleasure of eating and eating is one of life's great pleasures for people of all ages. So while your child enjoys an occasional soft drink with some chips, be sure that you have some better food choices like milk, flavored yogurt, whole grain muffins, dried fruits, nuts, fresh fruit, and vegetables handy for most other snacks.

Q *Should I feel guilty because my children drink a lot of soda?*

Your children are in good company. Studies show that soft drinks are frequently reported as the most liked food by teens.

A food consumption study done in 1977 and 1978 showed that soft drinks were the most frequent snack for teenagers. In fact, all Americans enjoy soda; in 1981 we each drank an average of 412 twelve-ounce cans. These drinks provide water, sugar (or artificial sweetener), perhaps some caffeine, and little else. Because sodas are acidic (have a low pH), if they are drunk in excess amounts they can wear away tooth enamel so that cavities are more likely. They also replace milk and fruit juice, which contain needed nutrients.

The caffeine content of soda is another issue. Many soft drinks contain some caffeine but the amount is far less than in an equal amount of coffee. Caffeine-free soda is becoming more available. See the chart Caffeine in Soda, page 141, and the question, "Is caffeine dangerous for my child" on page 138. We believe in taking a moderate approach. An occasional drink of soda will not sabotage your children's health. One glass a day would be a good limit. In fact, many authorities feel that moderate intake of soft drinks is better than some of the alternatives—coffee or alcohol.

Why not permit a little soda but at the same time be sure to keep a supply of milk, flavored milk, fruit juices, fruit ades, and perhaps some plain seltzer or more fashionable mineral water on hand for thirsty times.

Q *Is popcorn a good snack?*

Popcorn is delicious, chewy, satisfying, inexpensive, fun to make and eat, whole grain, and a good source of fiber. What a terrific combination! Popcorn can be prepared in a variety of ways from plain unbuttered and unsalted to sprinkled with grated cheese, mixed with nuts or raisins, dusted with seasoned salt or herb mixes, or coated with caramel. Something for everyone's taste, with a range of calories from less than

100 for 4 cups of plain, unbuttered popcorn to many times that amount for the fancier versions.

Children always have fun making popcorn. For the vegetable hater, a cup of popcorn can substitute for a less liked vegetable. The constipated child can be made more regular with a daily snack of popcorn—a high-fiber food. A child who is overweight can enjoy unbuttered popcorn as a filling, low-calorie snack.

Q *My daughter eats a lot of whipped toppings. Are they good for her?*

Kids enjoy these substitute toppings, as they are convenient and fun to eat. They love to squirt the topping out of the can or spoon it on a serving of pudding, ice cream, or cake. If used occasionally, they are all right. You should realize that they are not nutritionally equal to the food they replace— whipped cream. They do not contain the small amounts of protein, vitamins, and minerals present in cream.

A typical nondairy whipped topping lists its ingredients as water, hydrogenated coconut oil, dextrose, soybean and palm kernel oils, corn syrup, sugar, sodium caseinate, natural and artificial flavors, polysorbate 60, sorbitan monostearate, xanthan gum, guar gum, and artificial color. Homemade whipped cream usually contains only heavy cream and sugar.

While a 4-tablespoon portion of either homemade whipped cream or nondairy whipped topping has 56 calories, compare the nutrient content:

Nondairy whipped topping		Whipped cream	
Protein	0	0.4	g
Calcium	0	12	mg
Vitamin A	0	236	IU

As you see, the whipped cream has small amounts of some nutrients not found in the whipped topping. While the amounts in one serving (4 tablespoons) are not significant, eating large amounts of these substitute toppings is not desirable because they supply calories and little else.

Note: The remarks above apply also to nondairy creamers that advertisements sometimes suggest as replacements for milk on cereal or fruit. These nondairy creamers are not nutritionally equal to milk and should not be considered a substitute for it. A recent report tells of four children who developed kwashiorkor (severe protein deficiency) after they had regularly used nondairy creamers to replace the milk the children were suspected of being allergic to.

YOGURT

Q *My son loves yogurt and often eats it for lunch at school. Is this a good lunch?*

Yogurt is a good food and has all the nutrients that are in the milk it was made from. If he chooses a plain unflavored yogurt, it is exactly the same as an equal amount of milk, neither more nor less nutritious. It's likely, however, that he is eating one of the more popular flavored varieties, and in that case he would be getting more calories from the sugar, fruit, and other additions, and less protein, vitamins, and minerals. While an 8-ounce container of plain, low-fat yogurt has about 150 calories, 12 grams of protein, 415 milligrams of calcium, and 0.49 milligrams of riboflavin; 8 ounces of fruit-flavored yogurt has over 230 calories, less than 10 grams of protein, 345 milligrams of calcium, and 0.40 milligrams of riboflavin.

There are many kinds of yogurt available now and some have cream added along with sugar, corn syrup, and other ingredients that increase the number of calories and make the product more like a dessert. Label reading can help you compare yogurts, but even this can be confusing, as the container size varies from 5½ to 8 ounces.

Yogurt really should not be a meal substitute for a growing boy. It is not sufficient by itself. Instead it can be part of a more complete meal when eaten along with a sandwich or salad. If yogurt is the main part of his lunch, suggest to your son that he add nuts, fruits, raisins, or sunflower seeds to make his meal more nutritionally complete.

Note: There are many health claims made for yogurt, only a few of which have been substantiated. Yogurt will help to restore the normal bacteria to the intestine after antibiotic use, and yogurt has been shown to be effective when used as a douche for certain vaginal infections. Other claims about the benefits of yogurt have yet to be proved.

Q *Is frozen yogurt a good substitute for ice cream?*

Frozen yogurt is often considered a healthier low-calorie substitute for ice cream. This claim is hard to judge, as there are so many kinds of frozen yogurt available. A cup of plain vanilla frozen yogurt has about 180 calories (fruit-flavored types average 220 calories). Compare this with 250 calories in a cup of vanilla ice cream and 150 in 99 percent fat-free ice milk. These figures are averages, and you may find other brands that have a little more or less calories. The yogurt is really not much lower in calories than ice cream or ice milk. If you like the flavor of frozen yogurt, enjoy it, but choose types made with skim milk.

There is a new nondairy frozen dessert made with tofu (soybean curd) that tastes much like soft ice cream and contains 256 calories per cup. It is nutritious but is not low in calories.

CAFFEINE

Q *Is caffeine dangerous for my child?*

Caffeine is naturally found in coffee, tea, chocolate, and the kola nut extract used in cola drinks. It is one of the few common foods that acts as a drug in the body when taken in normal amounts. Two-hundred milligrams of caffeine is a pharmacologically active dose. This amount is in just under two cups of regular coffee or approximately four cans of soda.

Caffeine is quickly absorbed from the digestive tract, acting as a central nervous system stimulant. A "lift" can be felt within half an hour and continues for 3½ hours. The maximum effect of decreasing drowsiness and increasing mental alertness is felt in an hour. At the same time, caffeine acts as a strong diuretic, stimulating the kidneys to produce more urine.

Many of the side effects of caffeine consumption have been known for a long time—sleep disturbance; mood changes such as anxiety, depression, and irritability; heartburn; and stomach upsets. Further investigation is needed to determine the effect of caffeine on other health problems.

In the meantime, we'd recommend that you check to see how much caffeine your child consumes daily. The charts Caffeine in Soda, page 141, Caffeine in Chocolate, page 139, and Caffeine in Drugs, page 140, will help you. In the United States the estimated daily intake of caffeine by children is:

Age	Milligrams of caffeine daily
1–2	49
2–5	70
6–17	101

These average levels are safe and pose little harm to normal healthy children. Daily doses of 200 to 500 mg and higher can lead to dependence and "caffeine withdrawl" when the drinks are suddenly stopped. The symptoms—headache, irritability, nausea, vomiting, depression, drowsiness, and apathy—occur 12 to 16 hours after the last dose of caffeine.

Caffeine can be poisonous in very large doses. In one case, a small child died after ingesting 5,000 mg of caffeine in an over-the-counter drug. Obviously, caffeine-containing drugs should be kept away from children. Older children or preteens, who otherwise appear healthy but complain of jitteriness, fluttering heartbeat, or sleeplessness may be drinking excessive amounts of soda, particularly later in the day. For more information see the following questions, "Is there caffeine in soda?" and "Does caffeine cause hyperactivity?" on pages 140 and 221.

CAFFEINE IN CHOCOLATE

	Amount	Caffeine
Drinks:		
Hot cocoa	6 oz	5 mg
Cocoa, sugar-mix (water added)	6 oz	6 mg
Food:		
Milk chocolate	1 oz	6 mg
Semisweet chocolate	1 oz	20 mg
Unsweetened chocolate for baking	1 oz	35 mg
White chocolate	1 oz	Trace
Carob	1 oz	0 mg

CAFFEINE CONTENT OF DRUGS

Prescription medication	Milligrams of caffeine (per tablet)
APCs (aspirin, phenacetin, and caffeine)	32
Cafergot	100
Darvon compound	32
Norgesic	30

Nonprescription medication	
Anacin	32
Aqua-Ban	200
Bromoquinine	15
Bromo-Seltzer	32
Cope	32
Coricidin	30
Coryban-D	30
Dexatrim	200
Dietac	200
Dristan	30
Excedrin	60
Midol	32
No-Doz	100
Pre-Mens Forte	100
Prolamine	280
Sinarest	30
Triaminicin	30
Vivarin	200

Q *Is there caffeine in soda?*

Two million pounds of caffeine a year are purchased by
beverage manufacturers and added to soda. Most of the caf-

feine is found in cola or pepper drinks but other varieties contain caffeine as well—Mountain Dew and Mellow Yellow. Caffeine content must appear on the ingredient label, so it is easy for you to find out which sodas have caffeine. See the chart Caffeine in Soda, below.

Manufacturers are producing a growing array of caffeine-free cola drinks. The soft drink industry predicts that caffeine-free soda will account for 5 to 15 percent of the total soda market by 1986. They feel that young people want this type of soda. "The kids are rather tuned in to this [caffeine awareness] and are more nature- and health-oriented than I'd have guessed," said a Pepsi Cola advertising executive. Currently there are over 235 brands of soft drinks to choose from, many are caffeine-free. For more information on soda see the question, "Should I feel guilty because my children drink a lot of soda?" in this chapter.

CAFFEINE IN SODA

	Milligrams in caffeine in 12 oz
Sugar Free Mr. Pibb	59
Mountain Dew	54
Mellow Yellow	53
Tab	47
Coca-Cola	46
Diet Coke	46
Shasta Cherry Cola	43
Shasta Diet Cola	43
Shasta Cola	43
Mr. Pibb	41
Sugar-Free Dr. Pepper	40
Dr. Pepper	40
Big Red	38
Sugar Free Big Red	38
Pepsi Cola	38

CAFFEINE IN SODA (*continued*)

	Milligrams in caffeine in 12 oz
Royal Crown (RC) Cola	36
Aspen	36
Diet Pepsi	36
Pepsi Light	36
Diet Rite Cola	36
Kick	31
Canada Dry Jamaica Cola	30
Pepsi Free	12
Canada Dry Diet Cola	1
Like	04
Canada Dry ginger ale	0
7 - Up	0
Diet 7 - Up	0
Sprite	0
RC-100	0
Patio orange	0
Sunkist orange	0
Orange Crush	0
Fresca	0
A & W Root Beer	0
Hires Root Beer	0

ACNE

Q   *My son has acne. Is it because he eats a lot of choco-late?*

No, not really. Through the years, many different foods have been blamed for causing acne—chocolate, fried foods, nuts, shellfish—to name a few. Studies show that foods are innocent in most cases of acne. The foods that have been blamed and others as well cause skin eruptions only when a person has a sensitivity to the food. This sensitivity exists in probably less than one person in a hundred. Acne is caused by overactive oil glands and is most common in adolescence. More than 85 percent of all teens have some pimples at times. Some have a light sprinkling while others have more severe cases.

In some people with acne the condition is made worse by eating foods high in iodine. Some dermatologists say that excess iodine is excreted from the body by way of the oil glands in the skin. As the iodine passes through the pores it irritates them, causing pimples. Your son could try avoiding foods that contain a lot of iodine. He should stay away from kelp, iodized salt (and salted snack foods), seafood, and beef liver. Powdered protein supplements often have iodine added as do many vitamin/mineral supplements. Read the labels. Remember that iodine is not a factor in all cases of acne. Many healthful foods contain some iodine and if your son tries to eliminate all of them, his diet will be shortchanged.

Note: Acne is not caused by dirt, so constant face washing will not prevent it. Excess sun can aggravate the condition, as can moisturizers used too frequently. Coconut oil and cocoa butter, mistakenly thought to be sunscreens, are known to cause acne and this possibility is increased by exposure to the sun.

Q *Will vitamin A help acne?*

Doses of 50,000 to 150,000 IU of vitamin A have been prescribed for acne even though there is no proof that they help. In fact, rather than helping, large amounts of vitamin A can have a toxic effect, causing dry, itching skin, hair loss, headache, nausea, and even heart and liver abnormalities. A 16-year-old boy hoping to cure his acne took 50,000 IU of vitamin A every day for 2½ years. He developed severe headaches and nausea. To relieve the symptoms he had to have his spinal cord punctured to reduce the fluid pressure in his skull.

Acne has been treated with vitamin A acid applied directly to the skin. This is effective for some patients and does not cause the side effects which occur when large amounts of the vitamin are taken by mouth over a long period of time.

Recently it has been shown that a synthetic form of vitamin A (isotretinoin) can suppress severe acne when small amounts are given for short periods of time—15 to 20 weeks. Because of the potential for serious side effects, this drug is used only in very severe cases and then only after other treatments have failed.

OVERWEIGHT/UNDERWEIGHT

Q *My daughter is 12 and she is shorter than most of her friends. Will she start to grow soon?*

The growth spurt in the preadolescent period starts when the child reaches about 66 pounds. This weight represents a body composition of 10 percent fat and that is apparently a trigger to rapid growth.

The average age for this growth spurt in girls is from 11 to 13 years (for boys it averages 13 to 15). Your 12-year-old daughter falls within this age span and she still has time to grow. Her eventual height will be determined by many factors, including heredity and what she eats. Be sure that she eats well. Normal growth depends on a nutritionally adequate diet.

Q *My 12-year-old daughter thinks she is too fat and refuses to eat.*

Fifty percent of all school girls report being on some type of diet at some time. At any given time as many as 30 percent of adolescents are on reducing diets. Some may actually weigh too much—it is estimated that 30 to 35 percent of all teens are overweight—while some think incorrectly that they are too fat. During adolescence there is a normal increase in the amount of stored fat in the body. Commonly this fat shows up on the midrif and buttocks, making even a slim girl look stout for a short time. This increase occurs in girls aged 11 to 13 (in boys 12½ to 14½) and can easily be misread as the start of obesity.

Restricting food intake can be dangerous at a time when nutrient needs are great. At her age, if your daughter weighs more than she should she should aim to gain no more so that she will "grow" into her weight. For more information on determining your daughter's best weight and how to achieve it, see Chapter 7. If she is losing a great deal of weight and/or she is thin and says she is fat, this should not be ignored. For more information on this distorted body image problem see the next question, on anorexia nervosa.

Q *Can my daughter have anorexia nervosa if she is only 12?*

Yes, it is possible. Anorexia nervosa (obsession with weight loss) can occur as early as age 10. Its peak incidence is around age 14. It is believed that 1 out of 200 white girls around the age of puberty are victims.

Anorexia nervosa has been described as the "excessive pursuit of thinness" and is an eating disorder more common in girls than in boys. The name *anorexia,* meaning loss of appetite, is really not correct because some of the victims eat huge quantities of food which they then get rid of by vomiting, taking laxatives, or excessive exercise. They have a distorted impression of their body, believing they still need to lose weight even when emaciated.

A loss of 25 percent of body weight with no other physical problem is considered evidence of anorexia nervosa. Smaller losses are suspect if they are accompanied by other symptoms such as hoarding food, denying illness, overactivity, sensitivity to cold, absence of menstrual period, and growth of fine hair over the body. If your child has any of these symptoms you should see a physician immediately.

Q *Is anorexia nervosa the same as bulimia?*

No, it is not. People with anorexia nervosa severely restrict the amount of food they eat. Bulimic patients have frequent bouts of binge eating, consuming huge quantities. They follow this by self-induced vomiting or purging with excess amounts of laxatives to avoid gaining weight. In some cases, girls purge after every meal, others purge three to five times a week. It is very hard to convince them to stop this practice. We know of one girl with bulimia who ate a whole large-sized box of whole wheat cereal each day as a substitute for the three to five doses of laxatives she had been using.

An estimated 5 percent of college students (mainly women) admit purging. The actual use of this form of weight control is probably higher than 5 percent but the number is difficult to assess because many students will not discuss it.

Purging is not effective in reducing the absorption of food. A study has shown that even extreme purging, which produced 4 to 6 liters (a liter is a little more than a quart) of diarrhea, caused only a 12 percent decrease in calorie absorption. At the same time, the diarrhea can cause a loss of fluid and minerals that can be life-threatening.

PROBLEM AREAS

Q *How big a problem is alcohol consumption in adolescence?*

Most teens drink some alcohol. Studies show that 80 percent of all children aged 12 to 17 drink. Of these, more than one-half drink at least once a month and 3 percent drink every day.

About 25 percent of those aged 14 to 17 are problem drinkers, getting drunk at least once a month. Alcohol is particularly bad for teens who have high nutritional needs. Alcohol irritates the stomach lining, which reduces appetite. These "empty-calorie" beverages replace food and reduce the amount of zinc and the absorption of folic acid in the body. Chronic alcohol use affects the liver, which in turn reduces retention of vitamins A and B_{12}.

Q *Several members of the family have high blood pressure. Is there some way to protect my child from hypertension?*

Hereditary factors play an important part in the development of high blood pressure. A child whose parents, grandparents, aunts, and uncles suffer from high blood pressure is a likely candidate. Salt intake and overweight are also involved in high blood pressure. In fact, about one-half of children with high blood pressure are considerably overweight. Studies have shown that children who eat less salt have lower blood pressure. Research has shown that, as one would suspect, children get their salt-eating habits from their parents. Infants who eat high-salt diets continue this high salt intake into childhood.

It makes sense to help your child establish good eating and exercise habits now, as that will increase his chances for good health later on. This is good advice for all children but it is particularly important for families with a history of heart disease and/or high blood pressure.

Encourage your child to:

- Participate in some kind of exercise daily: biking, swimming, tennis, etc.

- Eat a variety of foods, especially fresh fruits and vegetables, starches (whole grains are best), lean meats, fish, poultry, and skim milk dairy products.

- Reduce fat, cholesterol, and salt.

- Maintain a good body weight.

- Avoid smoking.

It is recommended that children in families whose members have high blood pressure have their blood pressure checked routinely at their yearly school or camp physical. In fact, many experts recommend that high blood pressure detection be incorporated into all children's total health care.

Q *Is it necessary for my preteen son to eat a low-fat, low-cholesterol diet like the one recommended for his father?*

It would probably be a good idea. In the United States, children whose fathers have had a myocardial infarction (heart attack) have higher blood pressure and cholesterol levels than children whose fathers have not had one.

The reduction of blood flow because of deposits inside arteries is called *atherosclerosis*. It is a risk factor in heart disease and is believed to be worsened by high blood pressure and levels of high cholesterol in the blood. Atherosclerosis is found to some degree in all people. Up to the age of 10 it is present in the same amount in everyone throughout the world. But after 10, through age 15, atherosclerosis develops more rapidly in developed countries, where people eat diets similar to ours.

A worldwide study done by the American Health Foundation found that 13-year-olds who were obese had elevated blood cholesterol and high blood pressure. All of these risk factors can be reduced by diet changes, which is why it would be beneficial for your son to follow a diet low in fat and cholesterol and also low in salt. The charts Fat in Foods, below, Sodium-Rich Foods, page 150, and Cholesterol-Lowering Tips, page 151, will help you plan the diet.

FAT IN FOODS

High amount of fat:	Moderate amount of fat:	Low amount of fat:
Cooking oil	Whole milk	English muffin
Butter	Red meat	Bagels
Margarine	Eggs	Cereals
Lard	Cheese (mozzarella, ricotta, farmers)	Breads
Chicken fat		Fruits
Solid shortening	Cottage cheese	Vegetables
Whipped cream	Ham	Skim milk
Bacon	Frozen yogurt	Buttermilk
Nuts	Ice milk	Skim milk yogurt
Avocado	Muffins	Low-fat cottage
Cream	Corn bread	cheese
Salad dressing	Cheese pizza	Kefir
Mayonnaise	Graham crackers	Popcorn

FAT IN FOODS (*continued*)

High amount of fat:	Moderate amount of fat:	Low amount of fat:
Cream cheese	Waffles	Sherbet
Sour cream	Pancakes	Pasta
Sausage		Noodles
Cold cuts		Rice
Frankfurters		Tortilla
Cheese (Swiss, cheddar, American)		Pretzels
		Saltines
Ice cream		Matzoh
Cookies		
Pastry		
Donuts		
Olives		
Peanut butter		
Hamburger, fast food		
Potato chips		
Fried foods		
Chopped liver		

Note: Most of the child's food choices should be from the low and moderate groups, with occasional high-fat foods.

Sodium-Rich Foods

Kentucky Fried Chicken	Instant chocolate pudding
Big Mac	Canned vegetables
TV dinners	Tomato juice
Soy sauce	Salted nuts
Pickles	American cheese
Bologna	Potato chips
Frankfurters	

Cholesterol-Lowering Tips

- Use liquid vegetable oils (corn, cottonseed, soybean, safflower, sunflower).

- Choose margarine that lists liquid vegetable oil as the first ingredient.

- Limit use of beef, lamb, pork, and ham.

- Use only lean cuts of meat: bake, broil, boil, or roast.

- Use fish, chicken, and turkey.

- Use skim milk, skim milk cheese, and skim milk yogurt.

- Use more foods containing fiber.

- Limit eggs to one a day.

- Avoid nondairy creamers and whipped toppings.

- Limit use of coconut and palm oils, lard, and butter.

Part II

Nutritional
Needs in
Special
Situations

Five

Feeding During Illness

Refusing to eat may be one of the first signs that your child is sick. All children have bouts of common illnesses—fever, infection, colds, diarrhea, vomiting—that affect their appetite. For most of these illnesses, the child feels sick only for a day or two. You don't have to worry about missed meals during this short time. Appetites return swiftly and soon the child is eating more than usual, especially if you supply some favorite foods like custard, pudding, and ice cream. Annette always made creamy, fluffy tapioca pudding as a special treat for a child who felt "under the weather." Knowing this treat was available helped perk up the child's appetite.

Getting sick children to take enough fluids is another matter. It is vital that a child who has fever or diarrhea or is vomiting be given enough liquids to prevent dehydration. You'll find some hints on how to encourage your child to take these fluids in the questions and answers in this chapter. The hints will help you care for the child who is suffering from common childhood illnesses. Nutritional care is also important for serious medical problems, the treatment of which should be under the direction of your physician.

VOMITING

Q *What should I feed my child after he has vomited?*

Nothing at all for at least one hour. Just let him lie down quietly and give his digestive tract a chance to rest. Vomiting is the way the body gets rid of something irritating. It can happen from an infection, spoiled food, or eating or drinking too much. Some children may vomit as a reaction to a stressful situation. Whatever the cause, the result is the same. The child is left weak, mildly dehydrated, and low in some vital body elements—sodium, magnesium, and chloride. Some children develop severe gas pains after vomiting; this passes soon.

After an hour is up and your child has not vomited again, offer him a little water—sips every few minutes. If water stays down, you can begin slowly—very slowly—to add other fluids. During the next 24 hours give only simple carbohydrate foods like toast, gelatin, bananas, applesauce, cooked rice, or pasta and offer fluids. Ginger ale, cola (let these stand for a while to reduce the carbonation), grape juice, apple juice, and weak tea are good choices. Milk should be avoided at this time as it may cause gas and diarrhea in an already irritated stomach.

FEVER AND COLDS

Q *What do you feed a child with a stuffy nose?*

You may have heard the old saying that it is best to "starve a fever and feed a cold" but this isn't good advice. When a child has a fever, his body uses up extra calories and fluids; eating and drinking replace these. If your child refuses food, offer him liquids that contain some calories such as fruit juice or mildly sweetened weak tea. Herbal teas should not be given to a sick child because some of the herbs may cause side effects that could make your child more ill. When your child's fever subsides add some bland foods to his diet like custard, plain cereal, gelatin, bananas, applesauce, and plain or vanilla yogurt.

You'll often find that a child with symptoms of a cold doesn't want to eat much. In this case give him plenty of liquids and let his appetite be your guide. As soon as he feels better, he will eat more and make up for the small amount of food missed during illness.

Q *My child won't drink when he has a fever. What should I do?*

When a child is ill, often one of the first symptoms is loss of interest in eating and drinking. Although a feverish child is burning up more calories than usual, food is not the immediate problem. Most fevers last a day or two and as soon as the child begins to feel a little better he'll become more interested in foods. In no time at all he'll make up for the missed meals.

Liquids are another issue. Fluid intake is particularly important in a feverish child, as the increased temperature and sweating causes the body to lose more water. This water must be replaced to avoid dehydration, particularly if the child's temperature is over 100°F. Short-term fevers of less than 100°F do not require treatment.

Offer ginger ale, cola, Kool-Aid, fruit ades, fruit juices, iced tea, or water every 15 minutes. If your child isn't interested in drinking these, try freezing fruit juice or Kool-Aid into ice pops for sucking or into ice cubes which you can crush before serving.

Serve the drinks in fancy stemmed glasses and use a straw to sip. Put an iced drink in a small pitcher so the child can pour some out to serve herself. She can serve some to you too. Join her for a party of some liquid refreshment. Your company will be comforting to a sick child.

You should aim for about 4 cups of liquid a day for a 22-pound child, 6 cups for a 42-pound child, and 8 cups if the child weighs 66 pounds or more. Remember, if any fever lasts more than two days, call your physician.

Q *Should I give my child vitamins when he has a fever?*

Some experts recommend giving vitamin supplements to a feverish child because of the need for additional supplements when metabolism is increased. For each 1°F rise in temperature, the metabolic rate is increased by 7 percent (13 percent for each 1°C increase). This causes the body to burn up more calories, using more vitamins.

This increased metabolic rate is not a problem when the fever lasts only a day or two. If the fever lasts longer ask your physician if you should be giving your child a vitamin supplement.

If the decision is made to use a supplement, choose a multivitamin that contains no more than the daily requirement of vitamins and minerals. See Chapter 2 for suggestions on how to choose a multivitamin. Larger amounts of vitamins found in some preparations will do no extra good and may even be harmful.

DIARRHEA

Q *My child occasionally has diarrhea; what causes it?*

Almost all children have an occasional bout of diarrhea. This is not serious. Diarrhea is usually caused by bacteria or viruses. It can, however, be caused by excess intakes of vitamin C or products sweetened with sorbitol or mannitol, like "sugar-free" chewing gums, cookies, and candy. Even large amounts of naturally sweet foods such as apple juice can sometimes cause diarrhea. An older child may develop diarrhea because of excitement over a party or school play. Some young athletes have diarrhea on the morning of a big event.

A single bout of diarrhea really does not call for treatment. If the child has more than one soft, runny stool, see the following question, "What should I feed my child when he has diarrhea?" If the diarrhea persists for more than 24 hours or the episodes are frequent, consult your physician.

Q *What should I feed my child when he has diarrhea?*

A child who is suffering with a bout of diarrhea may not be hungry. That's all right. He can go without food for a few hours or even a day; just be sure that he has plenty of clear liquids. At least 2 to 4 tablespoons every 15 minutes depending on your child's size and age. He can choose from flat sodas, apple juice, grape juice, fruit drinks, weak Kool-Aid, weak tea, gelatin mixed with water, Gatorade diluted with an equal amount of water, or popsicles. Plain water is good, as are plain ice cubes. Each ice cube is equal to 2 tablespoons of water. Stay away from herbal teas. Although the tannins in regular tea can help curb diarrhea, herbal teas may aggravate the condition. Milk, bouillon, and soy milk should be avoided too. By the next day you can add simple, soft foods like bananas, rice, apple sauce without sugar, and weak tea (the BRAT diet) along with saltine crackers, dry toast, broth, carrots, and mashed potatoes.

From the third day on, gradually add regular foods to the child's diet. Milk and dairy foods should be withheld for several more days and then slowly introduced. Children often are intolerant to milk after diarrhea and it takes a few days before dairy products can be digested normally.

If the diarrhea persists longer than 24 hours, consult your physician.

Note: Some cases of chronic diarrhea have been noted in children who were eating a very low fat diet. They were given the diet with the hope of preventing heart disease when they grew older. When butter, ice cream, peanut butter, and whole milk were given, the children recovered in 3 to 10 days. This should serve as a warning not to put children on a rigidly restricted diet without medical supervision.

Q *I read in the newspaper that herbal teas can cause diarrhea. Is that true?*

Yes, some herbal teas can cause diarrhea and other unpleasant and even dangerous side effects. Many herbal teas, which are gaining in popularity as replacements for caffeine-containing tea and coffee, were once used as drugs and can produce physiological effects.

Tea made from buckthorn bark, senna leaves, flowers and bark, dock root, and aloe leaves can cause diarrhea. In fact, aloe is used by veterinarians to treat constipated large animals. There was a report of six adolescents who developed severe abdominal cramps and profuse, watery diarrhea three to seven hours after drinking buckthorn bark and senna tea.

Catnip, juniper, hydrangea, lobelia, jimson weed, and wormwood teas have been known to cause euphoria, hallucinations, and nervous disorders. Teas containing chamomile, goldenrod, and marigold flowers can cause allergic reactions in children who have hay fever or flower allergies. Comfrey tea, which has been recommended for 47 different ailments, contains alkaloids which can cause liver damage. An occasional cup is not a problem but frequent use may have a cumulative effect in the body. There has been a report of a woman who nearly died after drinking large amounts of comfrey tea. It was found that the tea was contaminated with a toxic herb. Herbal tea manufacturers are not always required to list ingredients and the tea may contain an herb that could have a negative effect on your child or yourself. To be on the safe side you should limit the kinds and amounts of herbal teas your child drinks.

Some herbal teas are safe and have shown no ill effects in people drinking them. These are Red Zinger, lemon balm, anise, rose hip, raspberry, and lemon grass.

CONSTIPATION

Q *Our four-year-old is often constipated. She may go a few days without a bowel movement.*

Parents often worry when their children do not have bowel movements regularly each day. Some parents were taught that daily bowel movements are necessary for good health. Their misunderstanding of stool habits may interfere with what should be a natural, routine activity. Just because your child does not have a movement daily may not mean she is constipated. Many children have normal stooling every other day or even every two days and they are not constipated. *Constipation* is the difficult passing of hard and dry stools.

If your daughter is indeed constipated, you can help her by increasing the amount of fiber she eats. Fiber is the indigestible part of fruits, vegetables, and cereals. Because it cannot be digested and absorbed, it remains in the intestine increasing the bulk (weight) of the stool, softening it, and helping it to pass more quickly and easily.

A small increase in fiber is usually all that is needed to

relieve constipation in children. Foods high in fiber are whole grain breads and cereals, nuts and seeds, fruits, and vegetables. Processing of these foods, such as peeling apples or potatoes or refining whole wheat into white flour, reduces the fiber content.

You can increase the fiber your daughter eats by making the following changes gradually. If you add too much fiber too quickly it may cause diarrhea or gas.

- Use whole grain breads and cereals (100 percent whole wheat bread, oatmeal, shredded wheat, Golden Grahams, Raisin Bran, Fruit 'n Fiber, Buc Wheats).

- Serve fruits and vegetables at every meal. Use juices only occasionally.

- Offer snacks of popcorn, nuts and seeds, fruits and vegetables, peanut butter on whole wheat pita, or crackers.

Try to have your child eat 5 to 6 grams of crude fiber daily, as this amount has been shown to relieve constipation in children. See the next chart, Fiber-Rich Foods, for other suggestions.

Try these changes for two weeks. If constipation is still a problem, add 1 teaspoon of unprocessed bran to cereal, meat loaf, casseroles, or muffins. Be sure your child eats at least one serving of the bran-containing food each day.

Setting aside 5 to 10 minutes at the time of day the child usually has a bowel movement is often suggested as part of a bowel training program. Some children, however, may find this procedure tension-producing and it may aggravate the problem.

Try taking a more relaxed attitude along with the diet changes recommended above. If the problem persists after three weeks, consult your physician.

Fiber-Rich Foods

These foods contain about 0.5 grams of crude fiber:

Apple (⅓ medium-sized with skin)
Applesauce (½ cup)
Banana (1 medium-sized)
Blueberries (¼ cup)
Bran (2 tablespoons)
Bran buds (1 tablespoon)
Bran muffin (1 three-inch diameter)
Broccoli (¼ cup)
Carrots (1 medium)
Corn (⅓ cup)
French fries (8)
40% Bran Flakes (⅓ cup)
Green beans (⅓ cup)
Orange (1 small-sized)
Pear (¼ medium)
Peas, green (¼ cup)
Pork and beans (3 tablespoons)
Popcorn (1¼ cups)
Prunes (5 medium)
Raisins (⅓ cup)
Raisin Bran (¼ cup)
Shredded Wheat (1 large biscuit)
Split pea soup (1 cup)
Spinach (½ cup)
Tomato (1 medium)
Wheat Chex (⅔ cup)
Wheaties (1¼ cup)

DRUGS

Q   *The package of medicine my son is taking specifies 1 teaspoon three times a day. Can I use a regular teaspoon to measure this?*

You shouldn't. If you use a regular household teaspoon you could be giving your son a drug overdose. Some household teaspoons may hold as much as two teaspoons. These spoons are not accurate for measuring. This is particularly a problem for children under 12 who may not be able to eliminate drugs as easily as an adult or older child.

One way to ensure that you are measuring out the correct dose of medicine is by using a measuring spoon or a calibrated measuring device available at your drugstore. This can be a cup, dropper, tube, or oral syringe with precise calibrations that mark off the amounts of medicine prescribed. Look on the drugstore counter, by the register, and you will easily find a children's "medicine spoon." A common variety is a hollow tube about 4 inches long with a spoon-shaped lip at one end so the dosage can be measured accurately and given without spilling.

Q   *Are there any foods my child shouldn't eat while taking an antibiotic?*

Many drugs, both over-the-counter and prescription, affect nutrition. Loss of appetite, nausea, changes in taste, upset stomach, and increased need for vitamins are common side effects. The table, Food and Drug Interaction, page 165, lists some commonly used medications along with their effect on food intake and nutrition. Some medicines are absorbed better on an empty stomach, and other medicines are absorbed better if there is food in the stomach. When there is a preferred time to take the drug, it is noted in the table.

FOOD AND DRUG INTERACTIONS

Drug	Effect on food intake and nutrition
Amphojel (aluminum hydroxide antacid)	Can cause constipation, decreased absorption of vitamins A and C.
Aspirin (salicylate)	Large amounts (1–3 g per day) can cause gastrointestinal bleeding, nausea, stomach pain, and vomiting. Absorption is slowed by food, but if taken with meals, milk, or antacids the chance of upset stomach is reduced.
Benzedrine (amphetamine)	Suppresses growth and weight gain.
Butazolidin (phenylbutazone)	Take with meals or milk. Usually not used in children under age 14.
Cleocin (clindamycin)	Take 1 hour before or 3 hours after meals.
Cortisone	May need salt restriction. Take with meals or milk.
Cuprimine (penicillamine)	Take pyridoxine supplement. Take 1 hour before or 3 hours after meals.
Cylert (pimoline)	Loss of appetite. Take after morning meal, give high-calorie foods 4–6 hours after drug is given.
Declomycin (tetracycline)	Nausea, vomiting, diarrhea, gas, and loss of appetite. Do not take with milk or dairy products.
Desoxyn (amphetamine)	Suppresses growth and weight gain.
Dexamil (amphetamine)	Suppresses growth and weight gain.
Dexedrine	Suppresses growth and weight gain.
Dilantin (diphenylhydantoin)	Affects folic acid and vitamin B_{12}. Vitamin D and calcium levels should be monitored. May cause upset stomach, appetite changes, diarrhea, or constipation.

FOOD AND DRUG INTERACTIONS (*continued*)

Drug	Effect on food intake and nutrition
Diuril (thiazide)	Use potassium-rich foods. Avoid food high in salt.
Ducolax (bisacodyl)	Take 1 hour before or after taking antacids or milk.
Erythrocin (erythromycin)	Take 1–3 hours after meals; don't take with fruit juice.
Flagyl (metronidozole)	Changes in taste and upset stomach. Take with meals or milk.
Furadantin (nitrofurantoin)	Upset stomach, loss of appetite, and nausea. May need to take with food or milk.
Gantanol (sulfonamide)	Nausea and vomiting. Do not give with food. Take with large amounts of water.
Gantrisin	Nausea and vomiting. Do not give with food. Take with large amounts of water.
Gelusil (aluminum hydroxide antacid)	Can cause constipation and decreased absorption of vitamins A and C.
Hydrodiuril (thiazide)	Use potassium-rich foods. Avoid food high in salt.
Hygroton (thiazide)	Use potassium-rich foods. Avoid food high in salt.
Isoniazid	Need pyridoxine (vitamin B_6) supplement. Take with food or milk.
Lasix (furosemide)	Take with a meal or milk.
Maalox	Can cause constipation and decreased absorption of vitamins A and C.
Macrodantin (nitrofurantoin)	Upset stomach, loss of appetite, and nausea. May need to take with food or milk.
Mineral oil	Take on an empty stomach or with fruit juice.
Mylanta (aluminum hydroxide antacid)	Can cause constipation and decreased absorption of vitamins A and C.

FOOD AND DRUG INTERACTIONS (*continued*)

Drug	Effect on food intake and nutrition
Mysoline (primidone)	Affects folic acid and vitamin B_{12}. Vitamin D and calcium should be monitored. May cause upset stomach, appetite changes, diarrhea, and constipation.
Motrin (ibuprofen)	Take with meals or milk.
NegGram (nalidixic acid)	Take with meals or milk.
Neomycin	Can cause lactose intolerance.
Penicillin	Upset stomach, diarrhea, may decrease vitamin K synthesis. Take 1 hour before or 3 hours after meals. Don't take with fruit juice.
Pro-Banthine (propantheline)	Upset stomach.
Ritalin (methylphenidate)	Loss of appetite. Take after morning meal, give high-calorie foods 4 to 6 hours after drug is taken.
Sulfasuxidine	Take vitamin K supplement.
Tums (calcium carbonate)	Can cause constipation.

Six

Dental Health

Since childhood we've heard that "sugar causes cavities," "apples clean your teeth," and "sugar-free gum is safe to chew." We believe these statements to be facts and repeat them to our children to help promote healthy, cavity-free teeth. Yet the average five-year-old in the United States already has had at least four decayed or filled teeth.

Many parents do not even consider dental care for primary teeth, taking the attitude that "they're only baby teeth." What they fail to realize is that loss of primary teeth can lead to malocclusion of permanent teeth, along with difficulty chewing and biting and the potential for speech problems. Abscesses or cavities left untreated can result in pain, chronic sore throat, and possible enamel defects in the permanent teeth that follow.

Although dental disease (cavities and gum disease) has many causes, it is largely a preventable condition. There are, however, many misconceptions about what constitutes good dental health. Why not test your own knowledge and see what you know about nutrition and the prevention of dental disease? Take the following quiz. Then read through the chapter to see how you scored. Some of the information you will learn will probably surprise you and will put to rest misconceptions you've had for a long time.

Nutrition and Dental Health Quiz

Circle the correct answer.

1. The connection between nutrition and dental health begins when a baby's first tooth erupts.
   True   False

2. Honey does not promote dental decay.
   True   False

3. Dried fruits are good snacks.
   True   False

4. Sweetened drinks cause dental decay.
   True   False

5. Apples and raw carrots help cleanse teeth.
   True   False

6. Peanuts and cheddar cheese stick to the teeth and cause tooth decay.
   True   False

7. Sugar-free gums do not promote tooth decay.
   True   False

8. Fluoride supplementation is important only during infancy.
   True   False

9. Eating a highly presweetened cereal for breakfast will cause dental decay.
   True   False

10. Ending a meal with a sweet dessert promotes tooth decay.
    True   False

Note: Answers appear on page 180.

DENTAL DECAY

Q   *What causes a cavity?*

By age 10, over 75 percent of all children have at least three cavities in their permanent teeth. A cavity is more than a simple hole in a tooth. It is an infectious bacterial disease.

Bacteria live in the mouth and throat of all children and adults. *Streptococcus mutans* is a common oral bacteria found in the human mouth. Interestingly, this bacteria is not in the mouth of infants before their first teeth erupt but quickly colonizes the infant's mouth once teeth appear. One theory suggests that parents pass this bacteria to their infants.

The bacteria are able to stick to the child's teeth by producing a sticky gel-like substance called *dental plaque*. Now the bacteria, firmly anchored on the teeth, ferments sugars the child eats into organic acids. The acids bathe the tooth enamel and begin to demineralize the tooth surface. The more often sugar is eaten, the more acid is produced and the attack on the enamel becomes a repeated occurrence. After many acid attacks, the tooth surface breaks down, the bacteria enter the tooth, and a cavity results. To prevent the cavity, plaque must be removed so that the bacteria cannot cling to the teeth, and the continuous supply of sugar in the diet should be reduced.

Plaque
with   + sugar = acid
bacteria

tooth
acid + enamel =   tooth
decay

Q *How can you reduce cavity-causing bacteria in the mouth?*

A clean tooth never decays. Some dental researchers have been able to reduce dental decay by 95 percent with a rigorous program of oral hygiene, frequent brushing, and daily flossing, coupled with regular visits to the dentist.

The future holds many other possibilities to combat the cavity-causing bacteria that live in the mouth. Some researchers are at work on a vaccine that could provide immunization against caries formation. Topical iodine solutions have been shown to significantly reduce the levels of bacteria in the mouth for long periods of time. Iodine treatments might someday become part of regular dental care. Dr. Hillman of Boston has suggested replacing the cavity-causing *Streptococcus mutans* bacteria with a strain of bacteria that does not cause cavities. His concept is that the "good" bacteria would fill up all those places where the "bad" bacteria are normally found and the cavity-causing would have no room to colonize.

Q *What is periodontal disease?*

This form of dental disease affects the tissue and bone that anchor the teeth to the jaw. Bacterial plaque allowed to multiply unchecked will eventually break down the tissue and bone surrounding the tooth. The plaque causes the gums to swell and turn red in contrast to the pink color of healthy gums. Periodontal disease is the major cause of tooth loss in adults.

Q *Do I have to worry about diet and dental health before my child has teeth?*

We can go one step further by saying that what *you* ate before your child was born will affect his future dental health.

Prenatal deficiencies of calories, protein, calcium, fluoride, iron, and vitamins A, C, and D compromise the development of the baby's teeth.

If protein intake is too low during pregnancy and early infancy there are changes in the structure, size, composition, and alignment of teeth. The child's teeth will not be aligned properly and will be more susceptible to cavity formation. When a pregnant woman suffers from iron deficiency anemia she will have a child more prone to dental caries. It has been estimated that routine iron supplementation in pregnancy and during infancy could reduce dental decay by 50 percent.

Once formed, dental tissue cannot change or repair itself. Tooth formation, if poor, is permanent. Tooth destruction by decay is permanent. Therefore, a good diet in pregnancy and good eating habits in infancy set the groundwork for good dental health throughout life.

Q What is nursing bottle syndrome?

Nursing bottle syndrome is a condition in which the infant or young child suffers extensive dental decay because the bottle, filled with a sweetened drink, was used as a pacifier, particularly at bedtime. A baby or young child should not be left with a bottle to be sucked on through the night.

At bedtime, as the sleepy baby sucks from the bottle, the tongue extends slightly out of the mouth and covers the lower front teeth. The sweetened drink bathes all the upper teeth and the lower back teeth. As the baby dozes off, active sucking and swallowing slows down as does the flow of saliva. The sugar in the drink puddles around the teeth, remaining in continuous contact with the teeth for hours. This sets up an ideal environment for the bacteria-filled dental plaque to produce acid and begin eroding the baby's teeth. We once counseled a child whose entire top set of teeth were so decayed and broken that dental surgery was required to remove all of the upper primary teeth.

The most effective treatment for nursing bottle syndrome is to prevent it by establishing good feeding habits in infancy, which include not putting the baby to bed with a bottle and not using sugar-sweetened drinks. If the nighttime bottle has already become an emotional necessity it should be filled with plain water.

SUGAR

Q *If my child eats too much sugar won't that cause cavities?*

We can't give you a simple yes or no to that question. What we now understand is that it isn't the amount of sugar that causes cavities but the number of times each day that the tooth is exposed to sugar. Remember, we explained: plaque plus sugar equal acid, and acid plus tooth enamel equal tooth decay. The more often your child eats food containing sugar, the more often his teeth are exposed to erosion by acid. Each time food sugar is fermented into acid, the acid attacks the enamel of the teeth for approximately 30 minutes. For example:

		3 meals a day	×	30 minutes of acid attack	=	90 minutes of acid exposure
	3 snacks a day +	3 meals a day	×	30 minutes of acid attack	=	180 minutes of acid exposure
3 cough drops a day +	3 snacks a day +	3 meals a day	×	30 minutes of acid acid attack	=	270 minutes of acid exposure

Sucrose, table sugar, is one of the most cariogenic (cavity-causing) substances in our diet. However, oral bacteria can ferment other food sugars as well. The following is a list of all the sugars that oral bacteria can use:

Sucrose	Lactose
Glucose	Mannitol
Fructose	Sorbitol

Substituting honey, molasses, or brown sugar for table sugar does not prevent cavities. Even children's medicines and vitamins may be in the form of a sugared syrup. Dried fruits and bananas, which we once considered good between-meal snacks, actually produce more acid than a doughnut that is not sticky and does not cling to the teeth. Sugared fruit drinks, which we frown upon because they lack nutrients, pass by the teeth quickly and are not cavity-causing culprits.

What does all this mean? Are we to throw up our hands, or better yet, throw open the cookie jar and let our children feast at will? Hardly! What we have done is to simply dispel some strongly held myths. The amount of sugar, by itself, does not necessarily cause cavities. The amount of times a day sugar is eaten is the key. The more often it is eaten the greater the acid-tooth exposure and the more likely it is that cavities will develop. See the chart Sugar in Snacks, on page 98, for some examples of food snacks that are high in sugar.

Carbohydrates, as starches rather than sugars—bread, cereal, beans, and vegetables—provide the bacteria of the mouth with less fermentable sugar and promote less tooth decay. In terms of the prevention of tooth decay, these foods would be better choices as between-meal snacks.

Q *Is it a good practice to let my children chew sugar-free gum?*

Sugar-free gums may be sweetened with sugar substitutes like saccharin or aspartame (NutraSweet or Equal). Neither of these substitutes causes dental decay. Other brands are sweetened with sorbitol and mannitol, which are sugar alcohols which are a chemical form of sugar and only half as sweet as sucrose (table sugar).

If mannitol and sorbitol are eaten between meals, when no other fermentable sugar is available, the bacteria in the mouth can convert these sugar alcohols to acid. If eaten as part of a meal (children rarely chew gum and eat simultaneously), sorbitol and mannitol are less cariogenic (cavity-causing) than table sugar.

Xylitol, another sugar alcohol, cannot be fermented by oral bacteria. The safety of xylitol, however, is in question because it has been identified as a possible cancer-causing substance in animals. It is currently under further investigation and not in use.

Another drawback to the use of these sugar alcohols is a syndrome known as *chewing gum diarrhea*. Chronic users may experience stomach cramps and diarrhea. In children, the incidence of diarrhea depends on the amount of gum or candy eaten in relationship to their weight. Two to three packs of gum (five sticks per pack) would be enough to cause diarrhea in a child.

Q *Do presweetened breakfast cereals cause cavities?*

If eaten as part of a breakfast, presweetened cereals are no more likely to cause cavities than any other food containing sugar in that meal. A test of breakfast cereals with 8 percent, 14 percent, and 60 percent sugar were all equal in their ability to cause dental decay.

There are a few possible explanations for this. One possible explanation is that oral bacteria may be able only to use a certain amount of sugar at one time. Excess sugar may not be fermented into acid. Another explanation is that when foods high in sugar are eaten as part of a meal, other foods might interfere with the bacterial action of fermenting the sugar to acid. Liquids drunk during a meal or saliva produced by chewing may wash away some of the available sugar. Foods high in fat (butter, salad dressing) and protein foods (meat, fish, eggs) interrupt the amount of acid formed.

If presweetened cereals are eaten throughout the day, as a snack, they will promote the formation of cavities. It is not the amount of sugar eaten at one time that is a factor in cavity formation but the number of times sugar is eaten during the day.

FLUORIDE

Q *Can fluoride prevent cavities?*

Most dental authorities think that the cornerstone of preventive dentistry is fluoride supplementation throughout childhood. Fluoride supplementation would eliminate up to 80 percent of all dental caries in primary teeth and as many as 40 percent in permanent teeth. During tooth formation, fluoride, a mineral, becomes part of the tooth's structure and results in a tooth enamel more resistant to decay.

Fluoridated water is the easiest and cheapest way to provide a fluoride supplement to children. When the municipal water supply is not fluoridated there are other ways to provide it. Toothpastes and mouthwashes are a source, as are topical fluoride applications performed in the dentist's office. Other more futuristic ideas are now on the drawing board: a fluoride pill that is chewed and swallowed, an aerosol spray which will coat the teeth, and a tiny device that could be bonded to the teeth or dental brace providing a continuous low-level dose of fluoride for up to six months.

Q *Isn't fluoridated water dangerous?*

More than 100 million Americans live in communities where the public water supply contains fluoride; however, not everyone agrees on the benefits of fluoridation. Opponents claim that in cities with fluoridated water the population suffers high incidences of cancer, cardiovascular disease, and Down's syndrome. None of these accusations has held up under careful scientific investigation. On the other hand, the relationship between drinking fluoridated water and the reduction of dental decay has been scientifically proved. Not only does fluoride protect children's teeth, but it makes the bones of older adults more resistant to osteoporosis (thinning of the bones).

When fluoride is ingested before the first set of teeth erupts (during pregnancy and infancy), it is incorporated into the tooth structure, making teeth more caries-resistant and preventing premature tooth loss. When fluoride is taken after the first teeth have grown in, the mineral washes over the surface of the teeth and stimulates remineralization. White spots on tooth enamel are precarious lesions that will absorb up to ten times more fluoride than healthy enamel. This absorption begins the process of remineralization of tooth enamel, preventing the eroded surface of the tooth from forming a cavity.

The end result of the use of fluoride is a significant reduction of tooth decay, by 60 percent or more. The prevention of tooth decay means less pain, discomfort, abscess, and infection for the child. The child's experience with the dentist will be more positive and less traumatic and the need for an anesthetic for dental work will be greatly reduced. In communities that have voted to stop fluoridation, there has been a return to a higher level of tooth decay and premature tooth loss within five years of discontinuing fluoride use.

In some communities in the United States, the natural fluoride concentrations in the water supply are high. Children in these areas develop teeth with mottled enamel that are extraordinarily decay-resistant. Their teeth, however, are spotted and not the typical "white" that is considered attractive.

Q *My toddler loves to eat our new striped toothpaste. Is that safe?*

There has been some concern about the possible excessive intake of fluoride by children who swallow fluoride-containing toothpastes and mouthwashes. Large amounts of fluoride can be poisonous. It is doubtful that a young child would take in this much fluoride unless he or she drank a bottle of mouthwash or ate a tube of toothpaste. Occasionally this does happen. We are apt to leave toothpaste and mouthwash within easy reach of children because neither is considered hazardous. Small children are attracted by the bright colors and minty flavor of these products and may swallow a large amount accidentally. Many mouthwashes, like Colgate's Fluorigard, contain warnings not to swallow and not to use for children under age six, unless recommended by a dentist. Even those mouthwashes which do not contain fluoride could be poisonous to a young child, as they contain a high percentage of ethyl alcohol (ethanol).

As parents, we need to teach our children how to brush their teeth properly and supervise the use of mouthwash. Some dental authorities suggest that a child be taught to use only a small amount of toothpaste, no more than the size of a small pea. Before the age of three a nonfluoridated toothpaste or plain water may be the wisest choice.

PREVENTING CAVITIES

Q *Is it true that when you eat an apple it acts like a toothbrush in the mouth?*

Many of us were taught that apples were "nature's toothbrush." Apples and other firm, fibrous foods were once believed to have cleansing properties that would physically remove plaque from teeth. Although this cleansing system functions well in certain animals, it is ineffectual in humans. Additionally, apples contain fructose, which is a sugar that oral bacteria can convert to acid.

Apples and other firm, fibrous foods like celery, carrots, and pears may not clean teeth but eating them stimulates the salivary glands and promotes the flow of saliva, which is important to dental health.

Even drinking water after a meal cleanses the mouth. Some school lunch programs promote "swishing" at the water fountain after lunch. Children are encouraged to take a mouthful of water, swish it around in their mouths, and then spit it back into the fountain. The children find it's lots of fun, and it helps prevent cavities.

Q *Do any foods prevent tooth decay?*

American children obtain a significant amount of their daily nutrients from snacks. Knowing this, dental researcher Dr. George Stookey at Indiana University is working to develop snack foods that are not cariogenic (cavity-causing). Ideally he'd like to develop a snack that is anticariogenic.

While we await Dr. Stookey's ideal snack other studies reveal that certain foods inhibit the tooth decay process or have a cariostatic (decay-slowing) effect on teeth. Often these foods inhibit plaque formation or plaque adherence to the teeth. Peanuts, sharp cheese (such as cheddar), and cocoa have these beneficial effects. These inhibitory effects suggest that the food that ends a meal can help to prevent cavities. A handful of peanuts at the end of every school lunch would help neutralize the 30-minute acid attack.

Now that you've read Chapter 6 you realize that all of the answers on the Nutrition and Dental Health Quiz on page 169 are false. You've also learned the three most important ways to prevent dental decay:

1. Proper daily brushing and flossing with regular professional care.

2. Use of fluoridated water.

3. Reducing the frequency of sugar intake each day and eating sweet foods within a meal.

According to Dr. Janet Brunelle of the National Institutes of Health, the number of dental cavities among American children is declining. Dr. Brunelle attributes this improvement in dental health to fluoridated water and toothpastes and to changes in dietary habits.

Seven

Weight Control

In spite of much research on the subject, no one as yet has answered the question of why some people get fat and others do not. Heredity, habits, culture, and psychological makeup all are factors that interplay to create the problem. What is known is that obesity left unchecked in childhood will be very difficult to resolve in adulthood. Prevention of obesity is far more successful than treatment.

The ideal time to start fighting baby fat is during infancy. Parents feel a sense of accomplishment when babies drain bottles or empty dishes. Young children are encouraged to join the "clean plate club" and food is often served as a reward for accomplishment or good behavior. These inappropriate eating habits result in a chubby child unless behavior is changed.

Most overweight children are not in need of a severely restricted or strict diet. In fact, severe caloric restriction may be harmful to health and interfere with growth. Heavy children need to eliminate poor eating habits and be taught how to eat sensibly. Their goal should be weight *maintenance* rather than weight *loss*. A child who is 15 pounds overweight should not be put on a diet to lose 15 pounds. He should be taught instead to maintain his weight because if he is 15 pounds overweight at age 9, by age 11 he will have grown into the weight with no weight reduction necessary.

Parents often are impatient with this slower approach to weight control in children. It is, however, the most sensible and safe method. Extreme caloric restriction or fad dieting at a young age may deprive a child of necessary nutrients needed for growth and development. Dieting further sets the child apart from his peers while it interferes with learning and decreases the ability to fight infections.

We have counseled overweight children and feel quite strongly that the weight maintenance approach, coupled with normal growth and regular exercise, is the most sensible and successful method. The tips, suggestions, and ideas we have shared in this chapter will help you to teach your child good eating habits. These good habits will help correct faulty habits that may have created a chubby child. If your child is of normal weight these ideas will reinforce good eating habits to prevent obesity in the future.

If your child is markedly overweight he should be under the care of a physician, nutritionist, and psychologist, so that all facets of the problem can be dealt with simultaneously. In the situation of a child under professional care the ideas in this chapter will help you to carry out the doctor's orders in a supportive and knowledgeable manner.

In other chapters you will find questions that discuss gaining and losing weight. Check the index to help locate these questions.

WHAT TO EAT

Q *My child tends to be chubby. What foods should he avoid?*

Eating is one of life's greatest pleasures. We don't believe in eliminating any one food or group of foods from a child's diet. If your child makes poor food choices, relying on high-calorie snacks and sweet desserts, he must be taught to eat more sensibly. The chart What to Eat, below, lists a large selection of foods with suggestions for frequency of intake. If your child needs to learn to make better food choices, he should choose items listed in the column, "Eat Frequently." As you can quickly see from the list, no food is eliminated. Sweets and high-fat foods are reserved for occasional eating. Your goal is not to deprive your son but to set limits on the frequency of his eating calorically dense foods like pastries, malteds, bacon, and candy.

WHAT TO EAT

Eat often	Eat occasionally	Eat once in a while
	Dairy foods	
Nonfat milk	Whole milk	Ice cream
Low-fat milk	Chocolate milk	Sherbet
Low-fat plain yogurt	Flavored yogurt	Frozen yogurt
	Cheese	Cream cheese
Skim milk cheese	Pudding	Sour cream
	Custard	Whipped cream
		Milk shake
		Malted
	Meat, fish, poultry, eggs	
Chicken	Fish sticks	Fried chicken
Turkey	Hamburgers	Fried fish
Fish	Steak	Bacon
Shellfish	Hot dog	Sausage
Tuna in water	Tuna in oil	T.V. dinners
Eggs	Luncheon meat	Spareribs
Veal	Egg salad	Duck
Cornish hen	Chili	

WHAT TO EAT (*continued*)

Eat often	Eat occasionally	Eat once in a while

Meat, fish, poultry, eggs (*continued*)

Eat often	Eat occasionally	Eat once in a while
Sardines	Taco	
	Pizza	
	Lasagna	
	Meatballs	
	Nuts	
	Peanuts	
	Peanut butter	
	Lamb	
	Roast beef	
	Pork	
	Liver	

Fruits

Eat often	Eat occasionally	Eat once in a while
Apple	Figs	Fruit packed in
Banana	Raisins	heavy syrup
Berries	Dates	Dried pineapple
Cherries	Apple cider	Fruit drinks
Grapefruit	Fruit juice	Fruit roll-ups
Grapes	Prunes	
Mango	Dried fruits	
Melon		
Nectarine		
Orange		
Peach		
Pear		
Pineapple		
Plum		
Tangerine		

Vegetables

Eat often	Eat occasionally	Eat once in a while
Asparagus	Coleslaw	Vegetables in
Bean sprouts	Pickles	cream/cheese sauce

WHAT TO EAT (*continued*)

Eat often	Eat occasionally	Eat once in a while
Beets	Sauerkraut	Fried vegetables
Broccoli	Tomato juice	Baked beans
Brussel sprouts	Vegetable juice	Potato chips
Cabbage	Potatoes	Corn chips
Carrots	Winter squash	Onion rings
Cauliflower	Beans (dried)	French fries
Celery	Peas	
Cucumbers	Lentils	
Eggplant	Avocado	
Pepper	Viandes	
Collards		
Kale		
Spinach		
Mushrooms		
Okra		
Onions		
Green beans		
Wax beans		
Tomato		
Zucchini		
Lettuce		
Romaine		
Escarole		
Corn		
Popcorn		
Tofu		
Radishes		
Chinese cabbage		
Bok choy		
Water chestnuts		
Alfalfa sprouts		

WHAT TO EAT (*continued*)

Eat often	Eat occasionally	Eat once in a while
	Breads and cereal	
Bread	Wheat germ	Sweetened cereals
Bagel	Raisin bread	Biscuits
English muffin	Graham crackers	Muffins
Hamburger bun	Crackers	Corn bread
Tortilla	Granola cereal	Waffles
Unsweetened		Pancakes
cereal		French toast
Grits		Cookies
Rice		Cakes
Pasta		Pie
Noodles		Pastry
Spaghetti		Doughnuts
Pretzel		Granola bar
Matzoh		Banana bread
Crisp bread		Cupcakes
		Coffee cake
	Other foods	
Mustard	Salad dressing	Gravy
Seltzer	Mayonnaise	Sauces
Broth	Butter	Oil
	Margarine	Candy
	Frozen ices	Chocolate
	Jam	
	Jelly	
	Honey	
	Kool-Aid	
	Pancake syrup	
	Molasses	
	Sugar	
	Regular soda	
	Sorghum	

Q *My child loves french fries. What should he eat instead?*

Although there is nothing wrong with an occasional serving of french fries, even for an overweight child, a lower-calorie selection should be used regularly. Below are suggestions for food substitutes your child may enjoy:

Avoid	Use
French fries	Baked potato
Mashed potatoes	Boiled potatoes
Potato chips	Unbuttered popcorn
Candied yams	Baked yams
Creamed corn	Steamed corn
Fried vegetables	Stir-fried or steamed vegetables
Creamed spinach	Steamed spinach
Apple pie	Baked apple
Canned fruit in heavy syrup	Fresh fruit or canned fruit in juice
Pastry	Raisin bread
Iced cake	Plain cake
Fried chicken	Broiled chicken
Fried, battered fish	Baked or broiled fish
Whole milk	Skim milk
Cream cheese	Low-fat cheese
Ice cream sundae	Ice cream cone
Fried egg	Hard-cooked egg

Q *Should an overweight child eat sandwiches?*

Why not? Sandwiches can be nourishing and filling as well as low in calories. They taste good too, and most children love them. Your child can select sandwich ingredients to make an interesting and tasty combination that is low in calories. See

Stack Some Sandwich Selections

Meat	Cheeses	Vegetables	Spreads
Chopped liver, 2 oz. (140)	Swiss, 1 oz. (104)	Lettuce, 1 leaf (1)	Ketchup, 1 tablespoon (16)
Liverwurst, 1 slice (139)	American Cheese, 1 oz. (93)	Tomato, 2 slices (10)	Mustard, 1 teaspoon (4)
Bologna, 1 slice (88)	Cheddar, 1 oz. (112)	Cucumber, ½ (7)	Butter, 1 teaspoon (36)
Boiled ham, 1 slice (66)	Cream cheese, 2 tablespoons (99)	Celery, ¼ cup (3)	Margarine, 1 teaspoon (36)
Deviled ham, 2 tablespoons (92)	Cottage cheese, ¼ cup (65)	Green pepper, 3 rings (5)	Mayonnaise, 1 tablespoon (61)
Dry salami, 3 slices (112)	Mozzarella, 1 oz. (80)	Onion, 1 tablespoon (4)	Miracle Whip, 1 tablespoon (68)
Spam, 1 oz. (87)	Muenster, 1 oz. (104)	Bean sprouts, ¼ cup (5)	Pickle relish, ½ oz. (21)
Bacon, 1 slice (45)	Cheez Whiz, 2 tablespoons (86)	Alfalfa, ½ oz. (5)	Steak sauce, 1 tablespoon (18)
Frankfurter, 1 (142)		Kidney beans, 3 tablespoons (60)	Barbeque sauce, 1 tablespoon (15)
Chicken frankfurter, 1 (110)		Avocado, ¼ (92)	Tartar sauce, 1 tablespoon (95)
Chicken, 2 oz. (166)		Carrot, 1 small (21)	Russian dressing, 1 tablespoon (74)
Turkey, 2 oz. (105)		Radishes, 2 (3)	Italian dressing, 1 tablespoon (77)
Roast beef, 1 slice (100)		Coleslaw, ¼ cup (28)	French dressing, 1 tablespoon (57)
Pepperoni, 1 oz. (139)		Scallion, 1 (9)	Peanut butter, 2 tablespoons (172)
Tuna in oil, ¼ cup (95)			Honey, 1 teaspoon (20)
Tuna in water, ¼ cup (63)			Grape jelly, 1 tablespoon (55)
Egg, hard-boiled (80)			Jam, 1 tablespoon (55)
Egg, fried (108)			Marmalade, 1 tablespoon (55)
Sardines, 4 (160)			

Note: Figures in parentheses indicate the number of calories.

Breads (Two Slices)

Bagel, 1 (165)	White bread (124)	Hot dog bun (108)
Cinnamon-raisin bread (120)	Whole wheat bread (112)	Hamburger roll (89)
Cracked wheat bread (120)	Pumpernickel bread (158)	Wasa Crisp bread (88)
Croissant, 1 (200)	English muffin, 1 (138)	Hero roll (400)
Italian bread (110)	Hard roll (109)	Pita pocket (90)
Rye bread (112)		

Note: Figures in parentheses indicate the number of calories.

the chart Stack Some Sandwich Selections, page 188. Your child could choose 2 ounces of chicken (166 calories) plus 2 slices of tomato (10 calories), with 2 teaspoons of Italian dressing (46 calories) in a pita pocket (312 calories) and make a sandwich with only 312 calories. Enjoy the sandwich with a glass of skim milk (90 calories) and an apple (50 calories). This makes a lunch of 452 calories which would be approximately one-fourth of your child's daily need.

Q *My seven-year-old daughter is chubby and drinks fruit juice all day. Should she stop drinking it?*

We recommend that overweight children *never drink fruit juice,* which may sound strange coming from nutritionists. We recommend eating the fruit instead. Think of how many glasses of orange juice your child could drink in the amount of time it would take to peel, section, and eat an orange. Eating the whole fruit slows down the act of eating and provides fiber which adds bulk without calories.

The following are some additional suggestions for what to eat to help your child control her weight:

- Eat whole grain breads and cereals and brown rice. They have fewer calories.

- For a spread on bread, use a half teaspoon of jelly or honey for each slice of bread.

- Cut down on butter, margarine, sour cream, salad dressing, and gravy. Serve all of them on the side, and use a teaspoon or tablespoon to measure them out to use less.

- Choose foods that require a lot of chewing—apples, unbuttered popcorn, shredded wheat, raw vegetables— they slow down eating and the chewing itself is satisfying.

- Eat foods that require a lot of work—nuts and seeds in the shell, unpeeled shrimp, artichokes, half melons, soup—this slows down eating.

- Avoid fried foods, which are very high in calories. Eat baked, broiled, poached, steamed, or raw foods.

HOW TO EAT

Q *Is it okay for my child to eat while watching television?*

For an overweight child, this is a bad habit. Often a chubby child must learn *how to eat*. The following are some suggestions that should be helpful to your child:

- Eat only when you are hungry. Whenever you feel like eating, wait 10 minutes before you take food.

- Stop eating when you can still eat a little more. Plan ahead to leave a small amount on your plate.

- When at home, eat only in one place. Never eat standing or walking.

- Eat slowly. A meal should take at least 20 minutes, a snack 10 minutes.

- Don't read, watch television, do homework, or talk on the phone while eating.

- Use a smaller-size plate (salad or luncheon) so that usual portions of food appear generous; eat with a luncheon fork and a teaspoon rather than larger utensils.

- Don't leave snack food around the house in inviting dishes. Keep all food in one room, out of sight, in the cupboard or in the refrigerator.

- Always eat three meals a day. Don't skip a meal to
  splurge later. NEVER SKIP BREAKFAST.

Q *How large should a child's portion be? My son
seems to eat large amounts.*

Serving sizes are standard portion amounts that you can use
as a guide. They will help you to feed your child the right
amount of food to meet his needs but not so much as to cause
weight gain. Adults often judge what a child should eat by
their own portion sizes. Inadvertently they may be overfeed-
ing and contributing to a weight gain.

Chapters 1 through 4 contain daily food guides for nutrient
needs developed according to age group of the child. You will
be surprised, especially for the young child, that standard
portions are quite small. Remember, children grow much
more slowly than infants or adolescents so they do not require
large amounts of food to maintain good health. Use these
daily food guides to adjust the portions for your overweight
child to help control his weight problem.

Q *My husband constantly nags my son not to eat so
much. How can I stop this?*

Your husband's intentions are probably well meaning,
though his approach is not the best. Kids normally react very
badly to nagging by parents. Often they do just the opposite of
what the parent is telling them. In your son's case, his father's
constant reminders not to eat may actually result in more
eating.

The following are some tips on how family and friends can
be helpful and supportive to an overweight child.

- Never mention weight, dieting, or food restriction to the child.

- Don't eat food around a child who is trying not to eat.

- Don't offer him food; let him serve himself.

- Don't stock the house with food your child is trying to limit or avoid.

- Don't cook or serve foods that are high in fat or sugar, such as fried foods and desserts.

- Encourage an exercise program.

- Don't nag him to lose weight.

- Don't blame him for being overweight or compare him to thin people.

- Praise him for his efforts to change his eating habits.

- Don't give your child food gifts or rewards.

- Give your child more time and attention.

EXERCISE AND WEIGHT

Q *Is exercise necessary for my overweight daughter?*

Most definitely! Many researchers believe that exercise is more important than calorie cutting for keeping children slim. In fact, children who are fat may eat slightly less than their classmates of normal weight. They remain fatter because they are less active. For lifelong weight control children need to be taught early in life the habit of regular activity. Team sports are fine because children usually enjoy them but they do not use up many calories. One- or two-person activities such as swimming, handball, and bicycling are more efficient calorie burners and help to control weight.

The charts Activities that Help Control Weight and Energy Used for Activities, below, will help you decide which are the best activities for your daughter. Remember, though, that all activity is worthwhile. Encourage your daughter to find opportunities to exercise. She could use stairs instead of an elevator, walk to school rather than take the bus, or ride her bike when visiting a friend.

Activities that Help Control Weight

Backpacking
Badminton
Bicycling
Handball
Jogging
Paddleball
Rope skipping
Rowing
Running
Skiing (downhill or cross-country)
Soccer
Squash
Swimming
Walking

AMOUNT OF ENERGY USED FOR ACTIVITIES

Type of activity	Calories burned per hour
Passive	
Reading, writing, eating, watching television, listening to radio or records, sewing	80–120
Light	
Dressing, personal care, playing piano, walking slowly, typing, playing pool	120–160
Moderate	
Light gardening, making beds, walking normal pace, volleyball	160–240

AMOUNT OF ENERGY USED FOR ACTIVITIES
(*continued*)

Type of activity	Calories burned per hour
Brisk Walking fast, cycling at 8 miles per hour, bowling, carrying golf clubs, doubles tennis, table tennis	240–350
Vigorous Calisthenics, singles tennis, swimming, jogging at 5 miles per hour, cycling at 11 miles per hour, waterskiing, cross-country skiing, dancing, basketball, football, field hockey	350–500
Strenuous Downhill skiing, running faster than 5 miles per hour, cycling at 13 miles per hour, competitive handball or squash	Over 500

Q   *Should my child weigh herself daily?*

That is neither necessary nor useful since weight fluctuates daily due to factors such as water retention, bowel retention, and time of day.

The goal in weight control for a growing child is weight maintenance, not weight loss. Many of the young children we've counseled are embarrassed about their weight and do not like to tell anyone their exact weight in pounds. In that case we ask them at each counseling session if their number stayed the same. If the answer is yes then weight maintenance has been achieved through good food habits. If the answer is no we ask if the number went up or down. If it went up we go over good eating habits once again. If it went down we empha-

One-Year Weight Record

Name _____

Age _____

Birthdate _____

Day of weekly weigh-in _____

Record the progress of your weight control program by coding your weekly progress.

____↑____ weight increased

____↓____ weight decreased

____M____ weight maintained

Goal: WEIGHT MAINTENANCE

Weigh yourself, no more than once a week, on the same day each week. Weigh yourself in the morning, right after you have gone to the bathroom. Wear no shoes and no clothing (a light pair of pajamas is fine). Record your weight and don't get on the scale again for at least a week.

Weeks	Weeks	Weeks
1_____	19_____	37_____
2_____	20_____	38_____
3_____	21_____	39_____
4_____	22_____	40_____
5_____	23_____	41_____
6_____	24_____	42_____
7_____	25_____	43_____
8_____	26_____	44_____
9_____	27_____	45_____
10_____	28_____	46_____
11_____	29_____	47_____
12_____	30_____	48_____
13_____	31_____	49_____
14_____	32_____	50_____
15_____	33_____	51_____
16_____	34_____	52_____
17_____	35_____	
18_____	36_____	

size that the goal is weight maintenance. Weight loss is not healthy for a growing child. Throughout this entire conversation, we allow the child to decide whether or not he or she wants to share actual weight in pounds. Let your child decide this also.

Use a weekly weigh-in as a guidepost to how things are going but don't put too much emphasis on the child's actual weight in pounds. The following is a weight record we often use with overweight children.

SWEETENERS

Q *Is there any harm in my 13-year-old daughter drinking diet soda?*

Diet soda is usually sweetened with saccharin or aspartame, the newest artificial sweetener.

Saccharin has been in use for over 80 years. It is estimated Americans use over 3 million pounds of it a year in diet soda. Recently, saccharin's safety was questioned as a possible carcinogen (cancer-causing substance) and the FDA (Food and Drug Administration) required that the sweetener undergo extensive testing. This testing period is still in progress but preliminary findings point toward a weak link between saccharin and cancer. In the meantime saccharin is available to the consumer.

Dr. Robert Hoover of the National Cancer Institute has voiced concern about the increased use of saccharin by children and adolescents, who consume much higher doses per unit of body weight than adults. Dr. Hoover has advised that "any use by nondiabetic children . . . and excess use by anyone are ill-advised and should be discouraged by the medical community." "Heavy use" as defined by Dr. Hoover is drinking the equivalent of more than four cans of artificially sweetened soda a day. See the chart Saccharin in Soda and Sweeteners on page 197.

Aspartame, a new sweetener approved by the FDA in 1981 and approved for use in soda in 1983, is marketed as Equal or NutraSweet. Made by coupling two amino acids (fractions of protein), the sweetener has no bitter aftertaste and blends well with food flavors. Currently it is found in soda, hot cocoa mix, Kool-Aid, gelatin desserts, chewing gum, and numerous other products. Some authorities have petitioned the FDA to proceed more slowly with the widespread approval of the use of aspartame. They cite animal and human studies in which aspartame caused chemical changes in the brain. More research is needed before it can be determined if the use of aspartame is a health hazard. In the meantime, we'd recommend using aspartame-sweetened products in moderation, especially for children.

Note: Some research has shown that people who routinely eat or drink artificially sweetened food actually take in more calories in a day than those who do not use artificially sweetened foods. Thus these foods may not be helpful in a weight maintenance program.

SACCHARIN IN SODA AND SWEETENERS

Soda	Amount	Milligrams of saccharin
A & W Diet Root Beer	12 ounces	126
Diet Pepsi	12 ounces	125
Diet Rite	12 ounces	144
Diet 7-Up	12 ounces	88
Sugar-Free Sprite	12 ounces	86
Tab	12 ounces	110
Sweetener		
Sucaryl Liquid	⅛ teaspoon	7.6
Sweet 'n Low	1 level teaspoon	20
Sugar Twin	1 level teaspoon	14

Q *If my daughter uses fructose instead of regular sugar will it help her control her weight?*

Probably not. Fructose, a sugar made from corn or found naturally in fruits and vegetables, is sweeter than table sugar. It contains the same amount of calories as sugar but because fructose is sweeter tasting, less may be used. The extra sweetness of fructose, however, is lost in many usual eating situations—in cake mixes, in hot liquids—so that more may be added, limiting its potential to reduce calories.

Some foods containing fructose are labeled *reduced calorie* because a food sweetened with fructose contains less sweetener, resulting in a product with slightly fewer calories. The effect of this calorie reduction depends on how much of the *reduced calorie* food is eaten and the calorie content of the other foods in the diet.

Note: Eating large amounts of fructose at one time may cause diarrhea.

Eight

Feeding the Junior Athlete

Recently a parent told us about a pep talk her eight-year-old son and the rest of the soccer team were given by their coach. "Don't forget," he said, "to eat a big steak before the game so you'll have big muscles." The coach was wrong on two counts—simply eating more protein will not build muscles and a heavy, high-protein meal is not the best pregame food. Also, good performance does not depend on one meal. Day in and day out good eating builds up nutrient reserves needed to support activities. In fact, the energy that soccer players use during the game comes from food eaten in the preceding week or two.

There are many misconceptions about food and sports. The young athletes, eager to build up their bodies and improve their performance, seem willing to try anything they hear might help—like extra vitamins, honey bee pollen, or steaks. Actually there is no magic food or supplement that will guarantee success in athletics. Good health habits including varied, nutritious foods and adequate rest along with practice and a stick-to-it will do well to improve performance. Many children will not be too happy to hear this but participation in sports can be a strong motivation to eat well.

The nutritional needs of young athletes are similar to other children their age except for the extra calories the athlete uses and the additional water lost in training. It is best if these extra calories come from carbohydrate foods like bread, rice, pasta, and potatoes. These foods also supply the vitamins needed for energy release. It is important for young athletes to cut back on these extra calories during times when they are not training and competing or they may gain too much weight.

Adequate water is at least as important as the kind of food eaten. Dehydration not only reduces ability to perform; it can be dangerous to life as well. This can be a real problem when there are workouts in hot and humid weather. Plenty of fluids are vital to the athlete.

NUTRIENT NEEDS

Q *Do athletes need extra protein?*

While it is true that athletes have more proteins in their bodies because of their large muscles, eating extra protein is not needed. Most children, including athletes, eat about twice as much protein as they need. This amount is plenty for even the most active athlete. Extra protein will not enlarge muscles; exercising them will.

With a high-protein diet, protein may be used for energy in place of carbohydrate, which is a more efficient fuel. This may be harmful because it increases the work of the liver and kidneys, which break down protein and eliminate its waste products by passing them out in the urine. Increasing the amount of protein may increase the amount of urine passed, which may contribute to dehydration.

Rather than worry about extra protein, the athlete should

be sure to eat enough calories. That way there will be enough calories to meet energy needs without diverting too much protein for energy.

Adequate, but not extra protein, and sufficient calories along with exercise will make muscles larger. These well-developed muscles will help the athlete perform better. Depending on your child's age, see the Daily Food Guide in either Chapter 3 or 4 as a guide to what your child should eat.

Q *Do young athletes need extra vitamins?*

No, they do not need any vitamins beyond what a good, varied diet will supply. Extra vitamins will not improve performance. They might give the athlete a false sense of security so that getting enough of the right foods seems less important. In that way extra vitamins can be harmful. They can also be harmful if very large amounts are taken, particularly of vitamins A or D. Large amounts of other vitamins are less likely to harm but neither will they give any benefit to the athlete. Young athletes should eat extra food to get all the calories they need.

Note: A condition called *sports anemia* has been described in athletes. This occurs in initial training when muscle tissue is forming, increasing the need for iron while at the same time there is a loss of iron through sweating. To make up for this increased need, more iron-rich foods should be eaten. See the table, Sources of Iron on page 78. Girl athletes who have begun to menstruate especially need more iron-rich foods.

Q *My daughter wants to know if sugar will give her more energy?*

Sugar, honey, glucose, and candy are considered quick-energy foods because they are digested and absorbed quickly.

While they do not help performance in short-duration sports like tennis, golf, or sprint running, they do help in long-duration events.

If your daughter wishes to use these sugars during a marathon or long bike ride, she should be careful not to eat more than 3 tablespoons in an hour, along with plenty of fluids. More than that amount can cause distention in the stomach with cramps, nausea, and gas. These can occur because excess sugar reduces the rate at which the stomach empties so that food and drink stay in the stomach a long time. Sugar also draws water into the intestine and may cause the body to become dehydrated sooner. This will reduce her performance and may make her nauseous. Sweets are best taken right before or during exercise because the exercise itself prevents an increase in insulin in the blood. High levels of insulin in the blood can lower blood sugar and cause poor athletic performance.

Q How much water does an athlete need?

Thirst is not always a good indication of need for water. Studies show that drinking enough water to satisfy thirst may supply only 60 to 70 percent of the water needed. It's a good idea to drink one to two glasses of cold water 10 to 15 minutes before an event and then 8 to 10 ounces of liquid every 15 to 20 minutes during the event. Cold drinks are preferred as they leave the stomach more quickly and also help to cool the child. More liquids should be taken after the event.

Some coaches withhold water during games. They allow the athletes to swish the water in their mouths but make the child spit it out rather than swallow. This practice is unsound and should be discouraged because water is essential during an athletic event. Withholding it could cause fatigue and mild dehydration.

Q *Do athletes need to take salt tablets?*

No, they do not. When a person perspires water loss is much greater than salt loss. In fact, when there is heavy sweating, the concentration of salt in the body is more than normal. Water is needed to dilute this intensity of salt. Taking salt without water, as in the form of salt tablets, isn't helpful because the body becomes even more dehydrated as it tries to dilute the salt to the same level as other body fluids.

Weighing will show the amount of water lost. Two 8-ounce glasses of water should be taken for every pound lost. Salt lost can be made up by the amount of salt eaten in regular foods and through extra salting of pregame meals.

If there has been a lot of weight lost during an event, 8 pounds or more, a weak salt solution can be given—⅓ teaspoon salt in 1 quart of water. In a preteen athlete such a great weight loss should not be allowed to occur. Gatorade or other sport drinks are not better at replacing salt lost through perspiration than this salt and water solution. See the question, "Is Gatorade a good drink for cross-country runners?" in this chapter.

PREGAME MEAL

Q *My daughter is in a three-mile race. Can any foods help her?*

She should make sure that she has stored maximum amounts of glycogen by eating high-carbohydrate foods for a few days before the race. Two days before the race she should

1. start avoiding gassy foods so she won't cramp.
2. reduce roughage (fiber) to avoid loose bowels.
3. omit salad oils, spices, and seedy vegetables to prevent diarrhea.

4. reduce or stop working out to prevent the loss of muscle glycogen stores.
5. eat nongreasy, bland foods like plain meats, vegetables, breads, fruits, milk, or juice.
6. eat more carbohydrates than usual, have four slices of bread instead of two at a meal.

Three hours before the race, she should have a high-carbohydrate meal similar to the one suggested in the question, "What should my son eat on the morning of a big soccer game?" in this chapter. Both protein and fatty foods should be limited. Remember that if there is any food she feels will help her to win she should have a portion of that food.

Q *What should my son eat on the morning of a big soccer game?*

Besides including a small portion of any food your son thinks will help him win, a good breakfast on the day of the big game could be comprised of oatmeal, toast and jelly, orange juice, and a banana.

The meal should be composed of mainly carbohydrates and eaten three to four hours before the game so that the food will have time to leave the stomach. Also, digestion of carbohydrate produces carbon dioxide which is easily excreted in the breath. It is best to avoid large portions of concentrated sweets as they can cause a stomachache and may lead to low blood sugar.

Fat should be limited because it stays in the stomach for a long time and it's hard to play ball on a full stomach. The meal should be low in protein because when protein is digested waste products are formed that must be excreted by the kidneys. Exercise limits kidney function so that these waste products may accumulate in the body and cause muscle fatigue.

Q *My son gets diarrhea when he eats breakfast before a baseball game. What can I do?*

Check to be sure that your son does not have a breakfast high in fat like bacon and fried eggs with buttered toast. Eating a lot of fat at a pregame meal can be the cause of his diarrhea. Fat also slows down the emptying of the stomach, which can cause cramping. It is best if all the food has left the stomach before the game begins. A low-fat meal will speed this up.

If any foods make your son gassy, do not serve them for breakfast on game days. Fruit juices, high-fiber cereals, and large amounts of fat and sugar may make some children gassy.

Breakfast should be eaten about three hours before the ballgame so that there is time for digestion and absorption of the food but not enough time for your son to get hungry. If this is not possible serve a small meal of cereal, milk, and bread without butter.

If your son gets very excited before the game, his excitement will interfere with his digesting any food. In that case a liquid meal might be best. Instant breakfast is good, or you can combine 1½ cups of skim milk with ¼ cup of nonfat dry milk, ¼ cup of water, 2 tablespoons of sugar, and ½ teaspoon of vanilla. This makes a nourishing, tasty drink. Liquid meals are also helpful for the child who tends to vomit from excitement before the game.

Q *What is carbohydrate loading? Is it safe for my 12-year-old daughter?*

Carbohydrate loading refers to a combination of diet and exercise which can result in the muscles' storing two to three times more glycogen than normal. Glycogen, a stored carbohydrate, is an important source of energy for muscles. This loading provides greater energy reserves and can be of value to the athlete who participates in long-distance or extended activities.

The procedure is started one week before the event. On the first day exhausting exercise is done to deplete the glycogen in specific muscles. On the second, third, and fourth days low-carbohydrate food is eaten, in other words the diet on these days is high in protein and fat. This diet is coupled with exercise. Then on the fifth, sixth, and seventh days, high-carbohydrate foods along with the usual levels of fat and protein are eaten. During these three days, training is decreased so that glycogen is retained in the muscles. This causes a temporary increase in weight as water which is heavy is stored with the glycogen—about 3 grams of water to 1 gram of glycogen.

Carbohydrate loading is not safe for your daughter nor is it necessary. For most athletes normal levels of muscle glycogen are more than enough to meet their needs. She can ensure this normal level by eating a high-carbohydrate intake every day and in her pregame meal. Spaghetti, rice, potatoes, and bread are high-carbohydrate foods.

More important, the safety of carbohydrate loading is uncertain. Because glycogen is stored with so much water, the muscles become waterlogged and may feel heavy and stiff, a liability for the athlete. It may prove to be unhealthy in the long run as well. Some authorities believe that carbohydrate loading damages the muscles. There have been reports of heart irregularities resulting. It may also be harmful for persons susceptible to diabetes, kidney disease, or heart disease.

Recent studies with trained athletes show that they can increase their glycogen stores just by resting and following a high-carbohydrate diet for several days before the event, a simpler procedure that is much safer as well.

Q *Is Gatorade a good drink for cross-country runners?*

Long-distance runners perspire profusely and lose a large amount of water and minerals from their bodies. This water loss causes fatigue and reduces the muscles' ability to work. If enough water is lost the body may overheat and circulation will be affected. Plain water is good to replace this sweat.

Orange juice, grapefruit juice, cola, and ginger ale diluted with 3 parts water (¼ cup juice or soda with ¾ cup water) is a good drink. Gatorade contains less sugar than these juices or sodas and so should be diluted with equal amounts of water when used by athletes.

Gatorade called a *sweat replacer* contains other minerals along with sugar and water, which are meant to replace minerals lost in perspiration. These minerals, while not harmful, are really not needed. The athlete has mineral stores in his body and can replace mineral losses with food and drink taken after the run.

BODY WEIGHT

Q *My son wants to gain weight quickly so he can make the football team.*

Many boys who want to gain weight fast eat large amounts of high-fat foods. It is true that fatty foods will provide more calories because fat is calorically dense. Weight for weight it contains more than twice as many calories as protein or carbohydrate. Although it may make your son gain weight fast, it isn't healthy and it may set the stage for heart disease later in life.

The best way to gain weight is through a consistent program of exercise supported by a nutritious diet of varied foods with some extra calories. This way your son will gain the weight he needs to make the team without jeopardizing his health. You should reassure your son that he will soon begin to grow much faster because at his age many young boys have not yet begun their adolescent growth spurt.

Q *My daughter is a gymnast and she is dieting constantly. Is this healthy?*

Whether or not your daughter needs to diet depends on her age, height, weight, and amount of body fat. Body fat can be measured with a skinfold calipers. Ask her coach to do this or have the doctor measure her skinfold at her next physical.

A growing athlete often may not have large enough reserves of body fat to permit a loss of weight. In that case, dieting results in a loss of lean body tissue (including muscle), bone, and fluids which can damage the body while reducing strength and endurance.

It is vital that a growing athlete get enough calories and nutrients to support normal development. Studies show that wrestlers who constantly dieted to reduce weight did not have normal growth during the wrestling season. They had catch-up growth after the season was over.

Note: Be sure your daughter understands that the use of laxatives, diuretics (water pills), or other means of removing water from the body are unsafe, do not cause permanent weight loss, and could result in poor performance in an event.

Q *Do sporting activities burn a lot of calories?*

The amount of calories used in exercise and sports varies with the size and metabolic rate of the athlete and with the

Activity	Calories used per minute
Climbing	10.7–13.2
Cycling	
5.5 mph	4.5
9.4 mph	7.0
13.1 mph	11.1
Dancing	3.3–7.7
Football	8.9
Golf	5.0
Gymnastics	
Balancing	2.5
Abdominal exercise	3.0
Trunk bending	3.5
Arms swinging, hopping	6.5
Jogging (slow)	10.0–15.0
Rowing	
51 strokes/min	4.1
87 strokes/min	7.0
97 strokes/min	11.2
Running	
Short distance	13.3–16.6
Cross-country	10.6
Tennis	7.1
Skating (fast)	11.5
Skiing, moderate speed	10.8–15.9
maximum speed	18.6
Squash	10.2
Swimming	
Breaststroke	11.0
Backstroke	11.5
Crawl (55 yards/min)	14.0
Walking	
2 mph	2.5
3 mph	3.5
5 mph	5.5
Watching television	1.5–1.6
Wrestling	14.2

intensity, frequency, and duration of the activity. Skill of the athlete also affects the number of calories; as skill improves, fewer calories are used. That is why the caloric cost of activities as listed in this table and others like it is just an approximate value. You can use this table to compare the energy used in various activities.

OTHER ISSUES

Q *What is meant by ergogenic foods?*

Foods like honey, wheat germ, and bee pollen are often called *ergogenic,* meaning that they have a special ability to energize the body. Many athletes eat these foods and supplements in the belief that they will get a little extra energy to help them compete more successfully. There is no evidence of any physiological benefit from these substances. However, if an athlete believes that a certain food or supplement will help him "win," he may be getting a psychological benefit that cannot be denied.

It is a fact that all foods containing calories supply energy, and 100 calories is equal to 100 calories whether they come from honey, bread, or bee pollen. Your body cannot tell where the calories came from. Eating these so-called ergogenic foods in small amounts will not hurt but there are more palatable and less expensive ways to get the needed energy.

Q *My son has slightly elevated blood pressure. Is it all right for him to lift weights?*

Isometric exercises like weight lifting and wrestling have been shown to increase blood pressure. These activities are not recommended for children with high blood pressure.

Other activities like biking, running, or swimming improve the health of the heart and blood vessels and are preferable for children with slight to moderate high blood pressure. For more information see the question, "Several members of the family have high blood pressure. . . ." in Chapter 4.

Note: Young boys do not benefit very much in the way of muscle building when they lift weights. This is because they lack a sufficient amount of male hormones that are needed to form bulging biceps. In fact children can actually damage their immature muscles and skeleton by lifting weights, and some studies suggest that it reduces growth in children.

Nine

Allergies

Food allergy has been recognized for a long time. In the first century before the birth of Christ, Lucretius commented "What is food to one may be fierce poison to others." In other words, one man's meat is another man's poison. You have probably heard this many times. By the 1800s it was recognized that asthma attacks could be related to food.

Any food could cause an allergic reaction. The most likely offenders are milk, eggs, wheat, peanuts, soybeans, nuts, fish, shellfish, and chocolate. Most reactions are to nuts, eggs, milk, and soybeans. If a person is sensitive to one member of a food family he may also react to other members. Peanuts are in the same family as soybeans, peas, lentils, chick-peas, beans, and even licorice. See the chart Common Food Allergen Families on page 214.

Most allergies are caused by antibodies formed by the body's immune system reacting to a "foreign invader." The antibodies cause cells to discharge chemicals like histamines, and these in turn cause the common allergic reactions. These reactions can easily be misdiagnosed because they are such common symptoms and also because sometimes the reactions are delayed for hours and even days after the food has been eaten. Canker sores and sore joints, which can be allergic reactions, may occur three to five days after the food is eaten.

Sneezing, itching, coughing, and runny nose are common signs of allergy but other symptoms can be vomiting, diarrhea, constipation, cramping, stomachache, nausea, headache, fever, eczema, frequent and/or burning urination, and even aching muscles. Some allergists believe that allergic reactions go beyond this long list. Hyperactivity, tension, fatigue, and emotional and personality changes have been attributed to food allergies. These signs may not always mean the child has a food allergy. In fact, a prominent allergist says that 20 to 30 percent of all the people who come to him for treatment of food allergies are found to be suffering from something else.

How do you find out if you are truly allergic to food? Sensitivity is established first by eliminating any other disorder that might be causing the symptoms. Then a comprehensive medical history is done. Foods eaten and reactions, if any, are noted. Skin testing is not a reliable way to test for food sensitivity in children. Using an elimination diet is better. For one week a very limited selection of foods is given which excludes the foods usually eaten. Rice and lamb are eaten because they are least likely to cause reactions.

Once put on an elimination diet, if the child has a food allergy, he is usually well by the fifth or sixth day. Then single food challenges are introduced, one at a time, for two days at a time to identify the offenders. For example, if a child is suspected of being allergic to milk, lots of milk and milk products would be eaten for two days as a challenge.

A recent study showed that only 35 percent of children who were believed to be allergic to foods actually experienced symptoms when challenged during an elimination diet. This shows that foods are often blamed for symptoms of allergies unnecessarily.

COMMON FOOD ALLERGEN FAMILIES

Food groups	Possible reactions
Milk (whole, dried, skim, buttermilk, cheese, custard, cream, creamed foods, yogurt, ice cream, sherbet, ice milk, goat's milk)	Indigestion, constipation, diarrhea, gas, abdominal pain, nasal congestion, bronchial congestion, sore throat, ear inflammation, asthma, headache, bad breath, sweating, tension, fatigue
Kola nut (chocolate, cola beverage)	Headache, asthma, indigestion, chronic nasal inflammation, skin inflammation, itching
Corn (corn, corn syrup, corn cereal, popcorn, Cracker Jacks, grits, corn chips, cornstarch, cornmeal, corn oil[a])	Irritability, insomnia, oversensitivity, restlessness, allergic fatigue,[b] headache
Egg (eggs, French toast, baked goods, icing, meringue, candies, creamy salad dressing, breaded food, noodles, egg substitutes, egg odor)	Hives, eczema, asthma, indigestion, headache
Pea family—legumes[c] (peanuts, peanut butter, dried peas, dried beans, honey,[d] licorice, soybean, soy flour, soy protein, soy milk, soy oil,[a] alfalfa)	Asthma, hives, headache

COMMON FOOD ALLERGEN FAMILIES (*continued*)

Food groups	Possible reactions
Citrus fruits[e] (orange, lemon, lime, grapefruit, tangerine)	Eczema, hives, asthma, canker sores
Tomato (ketchup, chili, prepared foods)	Eczema, hives, asthma, mouth soreness
Wheat and small grains[c] (rice, barley, oats, wild rice, millet, rye[a])	Asthma, indigestion, eczema, nasal congestion, bronchial congestion
Cinnamon[f] (ketchup, chewing gum, candies, baked goods, applesauce, apple pies and cakes, chili, luncheon meats, pumpkin pies and cakes)	Hives, headache, asthma
Artificial food colors (red dye amaranth, yellow dye tartrazine, colored foods, colored drinks, colored medicines)	Asthma, hives

[a] Only an occasional offender.
[b] Characterized by unresponsiveness, sleepiness, vague aching, weakness.
[c] Reactions to this group are severe, including shock.
[d] In the United States, honey is gathered primarily from plants in this family (i.e., clover, alfalfa).
[e] If the person is sensitive to citric acid, he or she will also react to tart artificial drinks and pineapple.
[f] Cinnamon-sensitive patients cannot tolerate bay leaf.

MILK ALLERGY

Q What is milk allergy?

Allergy to milk has been called the king of food allergies. It is the most common one at all ages and causes many different symptoms. Fortunately, after age one, these symptoms are not very severe and often may not even be recognized. One of the symptoms may be phlegm, the basis for the idea that milk causes mucus. It does, but only in sensitive people.

Milk is a mixture of water, protein, fat, milk sugar, minerals, and vitamins. A sensitivity to the protein (there are four kinds) in milk is the usual cause. About 1 percent of all infants are allergic to cow's milk. Breast-feeding is believed to help prevent the development of this allergy in infancy and later on as well. For this reason, cow's milk should not be given to an infant in the first year of life. Breast-feeding and avoidance of cow's milk are especially important if there is a history of allergy to milk in the family.

A child who has been found to be allergic to milk should avoid drinking all types of milk—whole, skim, low-fat, chocolate-flavored. Yogurt, cream, creamed foods, ice cream, sherbet, and cheese should also be avoided. Label reading of processed and convenience foods is a good idea, as many contain added milk, milk solids, nonfat dry milk, and dairy whey. Some children allergic to milk may have to avoid all these foods. Most children, however, have low-grade milk allergy and may be able to drink small amounts of milk.

Children who do not drink milk or eat foods made with milk need to have additional servings of protein-rich foods like eggs, meat, fish, and poultry. Adequate calcium intake may be a problem too, as milk is the major source. Spinach, broccoli, collards, tofu, and canned salmon and sardines eaten with the bones are all good sources of calcium. See page 124 for a list of calcium-rich foods.

Children are rarely allergic to the fat in milk. A small percentage of children may be unable to digest milk sugar (lactose). See the next question, "Is lactose intolerance the same as milk allergy?"

Q *Is lactose intolerance the same as milk allergy?*

No, it isn't, but they may be confused because they share some of the same symptoms. Stomach cramps, gas, and diarrhea are symptoms of both, but here the similarity ends. In milk allergy, protein, not lactose, is responsible for the reaction to milk and may include skin rashes and asthma as well as stomach upsets. Babies may be allergic to milk but they are rarely if ever lactose-intolerant.

People who are intolerant to lactose—and that may be as many as 15 percent of all Caucasians and 90 percent of all non-Caucasians—lack enough of the enzyme lactase needed to digest the sugar in milk, lactose. After the first few years of life, the amount of lactase produced decreases. The symptoms of cramps, diarrhea, and gas occur because undigested lactose absorbs water and is fermented by bacteria in the intestine, causing gas.

Children who are lactose-intolerant may have enough lactase to digest small amounts of milk, especially when it is taken with other food or is chocolate-flavored or cooked. Fermented milk like acidopholus milk, buttermilk, cottage cheese, and hard cheese may be eaten. Yogurt is also fermented milk, but the kind commercially made often has added lactose to give it body. Lactose is added to many other foods as well. Label reading is essential to tell if lactose has been added. See the following question, "What foods contain lactose?" for more information.

Note: A lactase enzyme preparation, Lact-Aid, is available and may be added to milk to make it more digestible. In some areas, Lact-Aid treated milk and cottage cheese is available. If the dairy products are not available, the enzyme preparation may be purchased from SugarLo Company, P. O. Box III, 600 Fire Road, Pleasantville, New Jersey 08232.

Q *What foods contain lactose?*

Lactose is found in all dairy foods—milk, ice cream, ice milk, cottage cheese, soft cheese, yogurt, eggnog, and cream. Smaller amounts are found in milk chocolate, hard cheese, and prepared foods like instant mashed potatoes, instant cereals, cake mixes, crackers, breakfast drinks, dips, and breads. Read the label to see if there is any lactose in a prepared food. Ingredients that tell you lactose is present include dry milk powder, nonfat dry milk, whey, dairy whey, and powdered buttermilk.

Lactose is even found in some drugs including aspirin, erythromycin, and the new sugar substitute aspartame, called Equal or NutraSweet.

FOOD ADDITIVES

Q *Do food colors cause allergies?*

Yes, they can. One color in particular has caused reactions in susceptible people. This is the yellow dye, tartrazine, also called FD&C Yellow Number 5. This color is added to many foods to make them look buttery, richer, or more appetizing. You can find it in gelatin desserts, cake mixes, cake icing, orange drinks, sport drinks (i.e., Gatorade), salad dressings, butterscotch candy, macaroni and cheese dinners, and seasoning salt.

Yellow number five can cause a stuffy nose and bronchial

asthma in sensitive people and it is estimated that one person in 10,000 may be affected. Those who are affected by aspirin may be sensitive to tartrazine too. This dye is now listed separately by name on food labels so that people who wish or need to can avoid it.

Drugs may contain yellow number five but since June of 1980, labels of prescription and over-the-counter drugs must list it when it is in the product.

Q *I have heard that some people have bad reactions to sulfites which are used to keep vegetables fresh in salad bars. Is this a danger for my children?*

It may be if they are sensitive to sulfiting agents. These agents have caused severe asthma attacks in susceptible people. Sulfites or sulfiting agents are often sprayed on seafood, fruits, and vegetables in supermarkets and restaurants to prevent wilting and discoloration.

If you are a label reader you may have seen sulfites—sulfur dioxide, sodium sulfite, sodium and potassium bisulfite, and sodium and potassium meta bisulfite—added to dried fruits, potatoes, and other products. Washing does not remove these additives.

These additives have caused acute asthma attacks in people who are sensitive to them, and it is feared that they may have long-term effects in others. Interestingly, sulfiting agents may even be found in asthma medications. It is estimated that as many as one-half million Americans are sensitive to sulfites.

The Food and Drug Administration has asked retailers who use sulfiting agents to have conspicuous signs, easily readable labels, or menu statements such as "sodium bisulfite added" or "sulfiting agents added to preserve natural appearance and freshness."

Consumer groups have asked that the use of sulfiting agents

in salad bars be banned and that these agents no longer be used on fresh peeled uncooked potatoes and in drugs used to treat asthma.

HYPERACTIVITY

Q *What is hyperkinesis?*

Hyperkinesis or "attention deficit disorder" (ADD) are medical terms for a disorder commonly called *hyperactivity*.

Hyperactive children, approximately 5 to 10 percent of all school-age children in the United States, have difficulty sitting still and learning. Even though these children are of normal intelligence, they have short attention spans, cannot concentrate, and are disruptive in school and at home. The majority of cases are noted at the time they start school.

Diagnosis of the condition is difficult and in some situations proper diagnosis depends on the observer. A study showed that older teachers were more likely than younger teachers to classify a child as hyperactive. Clinically, a child is diagnosed as hyperactive if he has a short attention span, easy distractibility, impulsive behavior, overactivity, and a positive reaction to stimulant drugs.

Q *Do food additives cause hyperactivity?*

In 1975 pediatric allergist Dr. Ben Feingold wrote a book called *Why Your Child is Hyperactive*. He believed that hyperactivity was due to the effect of artificial flavors and colors in foods and also to salicylates (aspirin-like components) which occur naturally in many foods. He claimed that 50 percent of his patients were helped by a diet restricted in these compounds.

The identification of salicylate-containing foods was confusing, as there were no accurate determinations. In fact, it is believed that there is probably some level of salicylates in all plants, including all fruits and vegetables. After a while Dr. Feingold singled out artificial colors as the main offenders.

Adherence to a diet free of artificial colors is very difficult. Luncheon meats, most ice creams, pudding, candies, and even nonfood items like toothpaste and vitamin pills would have to be avoided. Eating in school cafeterias and in restaurants is almost impossible. Of course, you would be able to plan a diet and lifestyle that can be free of artificial colors, and such a diet has no harmful effects. The question then is, "Is such a diet helpful for hyperactivity?"

On the basis of many carefully controlled studies, the answer appears to be that diet is effective in only a very small percentage of children, usually preschoolers. A recent study showed that in some genetically predisposed children, hyperactivity could be caused by red dye number 3, a red color now being used in place of both red number 2 (no longer permitted in food) and red number 40.

If a parent wishes to try the "Feingold Diet" there are Feingold Associations in many areas that can help you. Look in the phone directory. These associations are comprised of groups of people who feel that they have had success with their hyperactive children using the diet.

On the other hand, because the diet is not useful in the majority of cases, and because of the difficulty of adhering to the diet, parents should not feel guilty if they do not provide their hyperactive child with an additive-free diet.

Q *Does caffeine cause hyperactivity?*

Interestingly, caffeine was once considered a way to control hyperactivity. Further studies, however, showed conclusively that caffeine was not effective in the long-term treatment of hyperactive children.

More recent studies, done at the National Institute of Mental Health, have produced evidence that children who habitually consume several caffeinated soft drinks daily may experience the caffeinism seen in adults who drink excessive amounts of coffee. Symptoms of caffeinism are nervousness, irritability, restlessness, muscle twitching, insomnia, rapid breathing, heart palpitations, nausea, vomiting, headache, and anxiety. In some very sensitive children these symptoms may be triggered by as little as 50 milligrams of caffeine (the equivalent of one 12-ounce can of cola). Otherwise healthy children who show one or more of these symptoms regularly may be drinking excessive amounts of cola. Teachers have told us that many students report drinking soda in the morning before school starts. Their excitability followed by irritability, which interferes with learning, may be the result of a morning can of soda.

For additional information on caffeine, see the section Caffeine in Chapter 4.

Q Does sugar cause hyperactivity?

Many parents report that their children "act up" after they have eaten a lot of sugar. We feel that such an effect is due to something other than the sugar eaten. Perhaps a high-sugar diet crowds out more nutritious foods. Or was the child at a stimulating party where he ate a lot of sweets? Did he act up after an exhilarating session of trick or treating? Is the child overtired? Has a usual meal been skipped?

Recently, sugar has been shown to have a positive effect on learning. It improves attention slightly. Additionally researchers in Boston have found that sugar makes children and adults sleepy, not aggressive or hyperactive. It is obvious that more research is needed to clarify the effect of sugar on hyperactivity.

Q What is hypoglycemia and can it cause hyperactivity?

Hypoglycemia—less than normal amounts of glucose (sugar) in the blood—is often blamed for many symptoms—fatigue, inattention, weakness, headache, nervousness, hunger, trembling and sweaty palms, anxiety, and hyperactivity. Infants under one month of age may have this condition because of prematurity or an early developmental problem. A very small percent of these hypoglycemic infants continue to have the condition into childhood.

Pediatric hypoglycemia is not common. Most children who are diagnosed as hypoglycemic are prediabetic. The only reliable diagnostic test for hypoglycemia is called a *glucose tolerance test*. After fasting, the child is given a glucose (sugar) mixture and then blood samples are drawn several times to trace the amount of glucose in the blood. For a young child, this is an unpleasant and scary procedure. Before this test is performed, the physician takes a complete family history to see if the child had risk factors associated with hypoglycemia: premature birth, low birth weight, mother's toxemia of pregnancy, diabetic mother, or underweight for height. Does the child have a morning acetone breath (this smells like nail polish)? The child's symptoms must be evaluated in relation to the timing and type of food eaten and to the emotional situation. If many of these risks are present a glucose tolerance test would then be a logical next step. If the child's blood profile showed a lower-than-normal blood glucose (below 40 milligrams of glucose per 100 milliliters of blood) he should be treated with a high-protein diet, eating frequently throughout the day.

The popular press has exaggerated the incidence of hypoglycemia so that parents tend to blame this condition on school failures, hyperactivity, and undesirable personality characteristics. In the majority of cases this is not so. It's sometimes easier for parents to accept a physical cause for a behavioral or emotional problem.

Q *Do food allergies cause delinquency?*

You may have read about prisons where they are changing the foods served to inmates in the hope that less sugar, additives, and processed foods will decrease aggressive behavior. White flour, sugar, and food additives are the items usually controlled. However, psychological help is also being given and other changes made in the prisoners' life so that it is hard to tell what the causes for behavioral changes are.

Some researchers claim that 5 percent of prisoners commit crimes because of food allergies. This, it is explained, is due to cerebral edema (fluid around the brain) which causes restlessness, insomnia, anxiety, tiredness, poor motor coordination, and headaches in allergic persons. Many allergists doubt the existence of this condition as an allergic response to food. In fact, they believe that behavior changes are never found as the only sign of food allergy. The behavioral changes that occur are believed to be a result of physical discomfort.

Most of the claims that food allergy causes delinquency are based on anecdotal reports which are made when experiences from single cases or a few cases are described. Such reports are not meaningful in establishing evidence of a cause and effect. They do not meet the criteria for scientific research because the participants are aware of changes in their diet and have the expectation of behavior changes. Also the numbers studied were too small and there was no control group. In short, at this time there is no scientific evidence to support the claim that food allergies cause delinquency.

OTHER PROBLEMS

Q *Could my toddler be allergic to ice pops? She often gets cold sores after eating them.*

This is probably not due to an allergy but is more likely the result of "localized frostbite." This reaction to ice pops has been noted in a medical journal. There even is a proper term for it, *popsicle panniculitis*. The cold sores occur when the child keeps his lips on the ice pop or ice cream for a long time while enjoying it slowly. The lips appear swollen, dusky, and warm at first with blisters developing after a day or two. The condition is not serious, as the blisters heal quickly.

Next time your toddler has an ice pop, break off about one-half from the top so that the amount left can be eaten more quickly. This may prevent the blisters. Save the other half for a later time to be eaten with a spoon or have a treat yourself.

Q *My neighbor's child has celiac disease and is on a special diet. Exactly what is celiac disease?*

Celiac disease, also called *gluten-sensitive enteropathy*, is a lifelong sensitivity to the protein gluten, found in wheat, rye, barley, and oats. The allergy damages the lining of the small intestine and interferes with normal absorption of food. The child with celiac disease grows poorly. He may have frequent stools with high gas and fat content so that the stool floats on water and is difficult to flush down the toilet. Vomiting and gas are other symptoms.

The treatment includes a diet free of wheat, rye, barley, and oats that must be maintained indefinitely. In addition to the gluten-free diet, often the child may be temporarily sensitive to sugar and milk sugar (lactose). This is due to the damaged intestinal lining and usually disappears during the course of dietary treatment.

At the start of treatment, nutrient supplements of iron, folic acid, vitamin B_{12}, calcium, magnesium, and vitamin D may be needed. Once a gluten-free diet is followed, the intestinal lining heals and there is adequate nutrient absorption and no further need for supplements.

Recently, there was a report of Catholic school children with celiac disease who received communion frequently and had a bad reaction to the sacramental wafer. It is recommended that affected children eat only a small particle of the wafer to fulfill this religious practice.

Further information about celiac disease is available from Celiac Society of U.S.A., 45 Glifford Ave., Jersey City, New Jersey 07304.

Part III

Kid-Tested
Recipes

There are very few children who will eat every food. The recipes we included, however, will appeal to most children. The selections are not all-inclusive. There are many good cookbooks that can give you additional ideas. We tried only to give you a few good recipes that are easy to prepare and most likely to be eaten. Many of the recipes are for items we suggested in earlier chapters. Vegetables are obvious by their omission.

As we've said before, it has been our experience that those cooked vegetables children enjoy are usually simply prepared by stir-frying or steaming. Most prefer raw vegetables, salad, or fruit. The main dish recipes we've suggested could be served with a plain or raw vegetable, a salad, or fresh fruit to round out the meal.

All of these recipes can be prepared by preteens and many could be cooked successfully by younger children. Children who help with cooking enjoy eating and are more willing to try a new food. Teaching children basic cooking skills and kitchen safety helps to build confidence and self-reliance and increases eating enjoyment.

Standard Abbreviations

t. = teaspoon	qt. = quart
T. = tablespoon	oz. = ounce
c. = cup	lb. = pound
pt. = pint	

Equivalent Measures

1 tablespoon = 3 teaspoons	¼ cup = 2 ounces
4 tablespoons = ¼ cup	¼ cup = 4 ounces
8 tablespoons = ½ cup	¾ cup = 6 ounces
12 tablespoons = ¾ cup	1 cup = 8 ounces
16 tablespoons = 1 cup	2 cups = 1 pint or 16 ounces
2 tablespoons = 1 ounce	4 cups = 1 quart or
	2 pints or
	32 ounces

How to Follow a Recipe

1. Read it through.
2. Assemble all ingredients.
3. Measure all ingredients.
4. Proceed with instructions.

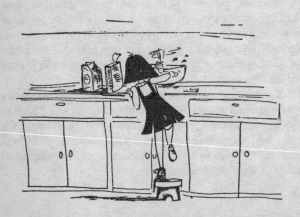

MEALTIME IDEAS

Skillet Rice Dinner

Yield: 4 servings

    1 T. oil
    ½ c. chopped celery
    1 medium onion, diced
    2 cloves garlic, chopped
    ½ lb. chopped beef
    ½ c. regular rice
    1 can (1 lb.) stewed tomatoes
    ¼ c. water
    3 T. grated Parmesan cheese (optional)

In a 10-inch skillet heat oil; saute celery, onion, and garlic until soft but not brown; add beef and saute until meat loses its pink color. Add rice, tomatoes, and water; stir to combine thoroughly. Cover skillet and simmer 25 minutes or until rice is tender.
Sprinkle with cheese, cover, and continue to cook until cheese is melted, about 3 minutes.

Pocket Salad Sandwich

    1 whole wheat pita pocket bread
    1 T. favorite salad dressing
    Favorite filling*

Cut approximately 2 inches off one edge of pocket bread; stuff with filling or mixture of fillings; drizzle with dressing; serve.

* suggested fillings:

Shredded lettuce	Chopped egg
Sliced avocado	Flaked tuna
Grated carrots	Diced, cooked chicken
Sliced olives	Julienne ham
Bean sprout	Grated cheese
Sliced cucumber	Cottage cheese
Sliced apple	Cold, cooked beans
Raisins	Any leftovers
Nuts	
Chopped green onions	
Sesame seeds	
Sliced tomato	
Sunflower seeds	

Macaroni Squares

Yield: 4 servings

¾ c. elbow macaroni
1 medium onion, diced
2 T. butter or margarine
3 eggs, slightly beaten
¾ c. skim milk
2 T. grated Parmesan cheese
or
½ c. grated cheddar or Swiss cheese
Paprika

Cook elbow macaroni according to package directions; drain.
In a small skillet saute onion in butter until soft and transparent.
In a bowl combine macaroni, onion, and all remaining ingredients; stir to combine.
Spoon macaroni mixture into a greased 8- by 8-inch baking dish; sprinkle lightly with paprika.
Bake 30 minutes at 325°F. Cut into four squares to serve.

Create-a-Quiche

Yield: 6 small or 4 generous servings

1 unbaked (9-inch) pie shell
¾ c. shredded cheese*
¾ c. meat, poultry, seafood, or vegetable, cooked and cut in
small pieces†
6 large eggs, beaten
1¼ c. skim milk
¼ t. dried parsley or 1 T. fresh parsley, chopped
⅛ t. pepper

---

* Any cheese may be used; if Parmesan or hard grating cheese is used reduce amount to ¼ c.
† Filling suggestions: cooked, crumbled bacon; cooked, drained sausage; cooked, drained ground beef; diced ham; cooked, diced chicken; cooked shrimp; flaked crab; flaked salmon; sauteed mushrooms; sauteed onions; sauteed broccoli; cooked chopped asparagus spears; cooked chopped spinach; cooked mixed vegetables.

Sprinkle cheese and filling (meat, poultry, seafood, or vegetable) into pie shell.

Combine eggs, milk, parsley, and pepper, and pour over filling in pie shell.

Bake at 375°F for 35 to 40 minutes. Let stand 5 minutes before cutting into wedges.

Pizza Scramble

Yield: 2 servings

   2 T. vegetable oil
   4 large eggs
   2 T. water
   ⅛ t. dried oregano
   ¼ c. pizza sauce or tomato sauce
   ¼ c. grated mozzarella cheese
   1 t. grated Parmesan cheese

Heat oil in an 8-inch skillet.

Combine eggs, water, and oregano; pour into hot skillet; reduce heat to medium and scramble eggs until firm but moist; reduce heat to low.

Spoon sauce over egg mixture, top with cheese; cover skillet and continue to cook for 5 minutes or until cheese is melted and sauce is hot. Cut in half and serve immediately.

Welsh Rarebit

Serves: 4 toddlers
*   2 children*

   1 c. grated cheese (any variety will work)
   ½ c. milk
   ½ t. prepared mustard
   4 slices whole wheat toast cut in wedges

Combine all ingredients, except toast, in a small saucepan; heat, stirring constantly over low heat until cheese is completely melted and mixture is smooth.

Serve immediately over toast wedges.

VEGETABLES

Stir-Fry Vegetables

Yield: 6 servings

2 T. oil
4–6 cloves of garlic, sliced
1 large onion, sliced
3 c. raw fresh vegetable, cut up*
1 t. molasses
1 t. soy sauce

Heat oil in a large skillet; stir-fry garlic and onions until soft; add
remaining vegetables and stir-fry 5 to 7 minutes or until crisp tender.
Add molasses and soy sauce; stir to blend flavors, serve.

* Use any one or combination of the following: broccoli, cauliflower, cabbage,
mushrooms, zucchini, summer squash, bean sprouts (cook only 1 minute), spinach.

Cabbage and Noodles

Yield: 6 servings

4 oz. egg noodles
3 T. butter or margarine
3 c. shredded cabbage
Paprika, to taste

Cook noodles, according to package directions, drain, rinse.
Melt butter in a skillet; add cabbage and stir-fry until soft but crisp
tender.
Add cooked noodles to cabbage and heat over a low flame 3 to 5
minutes.
Serve hot.

Corny Cornbread

Yield: 6 servings

1¼ c. yellow cornmeal
1 t. baking powder

2 eggs
1 can (8 oz.) creamed corn
1 c. (8 oz.) vanilla yogurt
3 T. butter or margarine, melted

Combine all ingredients; mix thoroughly.
Spoon mixture into a greased 8-inch square baking pan.
Bake 25 minutes at 375°F.

PANCAKES AND CEREAL

Whole Wheat Pancakes

Yield: Twelve 6-inch pancakes

¼ c. wheat germ
2 c. whole wheat flour
2 t. baking powder
1 T. brown sugar
2 large eggs, slightly beaten
2½ c. skim milk
2 T. oil

Combine all dry ingredients.
Combine eggs and milk.
Add milk mixture to flour mixture and beat thoroughly to combine; stir in oil.
Heat griddle but do not grease. Griddle should be so hot that when you sprinkle a few drops of water on surface, they dance.
Pour batter onto griddle, approximately ½ cup per pancake.
Bake pancake, over medium heat, turning when bubbles come to the surface and pop and edges are slightly dry.
To freeze; Make pancakes and cool; place on a tray or cookie sheet in a single layer; freeze about 1 hour or until firmly frozen; wrap each pancake and place wrapped pancakes in a plastic bag. Return to freezer; use as needed.
To reheat: Unwrap pancake, place frozen pancake on a cookie sheet and heat 5 to 7 minutes at 350°F.

Whole wheat pancakes are more flavorful than those made with white flour, therefore, they can be used in ways not usually considered "traditional" pancake meals. Preteens may have a pancake roll-up as an after-school snack. Preschoolers will enjoy them for lunch. The whole family can eat them for a quick dinner. Try some of the following suggestions combined with a fresh fruit salad and you'll have a nutritious and quick meal:

Pancake Roll-Ups

Fill the pancake with suggested filling, roll up, and eat with fingers or fork.

- Ham and cheese pancakes: layer one slice ham and one slice cheese over hot pancake; roll to serve.

- Apple-cheese pancake: spread a thin layer of whipped cream cheese and then a thin layer of apple sauce; roll to serve.

- Egg roll-up: layer a pancake with a scrambled egg; roll and serve.

- Creamy chicken roll-up: spread approximately ¼ cup creamed chicken over pancake; roll to serve.

- Fruit pancake: spread stewed dried fruit over pancake; roll to serve.

Granola is a high-protein cereal product made from natural grain products. Granola, a generic name for a variety of mixtures, might include rolled oats, honey, wheat germ, nuts, and dried fruit. Crunchy granola originated in California.

Crunchy Granola

Yield: 6 cups

⅔ c. wheat germ
1 T. sesame seeds
¼ c. raisins or cut up dried fruit
2 c. rolled oats
2 c. rolled wheat (wheat flakes)
⅓ c. melted margarine or butter
½ c. brown sugar
¼ c. shredded coconut (optional)
¼ c. chopped nuts

Combine wheat germ, sesame seeds, and dried fruit; spread in a shallow baking pan and toast for 15 minutes at 200°F. Set aside to cool.
Combine rolled oats, rolled wheat, melted margarine, brown sugar, coconut, and nuts; spread in a shallow baking pan and bake for 45 minutes at 250°F, stirring occasionally. Cool.
When both mixtures are cool, combine and store in a tightly covered container. Crunchy Granola will remain fresh up to 4 months.

DRINKS

These cool drinks are good substitutes for less nutritious colas or carbonated sodas. They are a good meal accompaniment or snack drink.

Fruit Shake

Yield: 2 servings

1 large banana, peeled and cut in large chunks
1 c. skim milk
1 can (6 oz.) unsweetened pineapple juice

Combine all ingredients in a blender container and blend until combined and frothy.
Serve immediately.

Create-a-Soda

Yield: 1 serving

> ⅔ c. fruit juice (any variety)
> ⅓ c. seltzer
> 2–3 ice cubes

Combine in a large glass and serve.

Nectar Cooler

Yield: 1 serving

> ⅓ c. fruit nectar (any variety)
> ⅔ c. seltzer
> 1 orange wedge
> 2–3 ice cubes

Combine in a large glass and serve.

Orange Julius

Yield: 4 servings

> 1 can (6 oz.) frozen concentrated orange juice
> 1¾ c. water
> ½ c. nonfat dry milk powder
> 1 t. vanilla
> 3 T. honey
> 12 ice cubes

Combine all ingredients in a blender container, and blend until combined and frothy.
Serve immediately.

SNACKS

Annette's Mandelbrot Cookies

Yield: 2½ dozen large cookies

    2 c. regular flour
    ¾ c. whole wheat flour
    ¾ c. sugar
    2½ t. baking powder
    1 c. chocolate chips
    ½ c. chopped walnuts
    6 T. oil
    3 eggs, slightly beaten
    ½ t. vanilla

Combine first six ingredients; add oil, eggs, and vanilla; mix to combine thoroughly.

Divide dough in half; grease your hands well and shape each half of dough into a log 2 inches wide and 14 inches long. Place the two logs on a greased cookie sheet.

Bake 30 minutes at 350°F. Turn off oven. Cool 5 minutes and cut logs into 1-inch slices. Lay sliced cookies on their sides and return to warm oven for 5 to 7 minutes to toast lightly, if you wish.

Ice Pops

Yield: 8 ice pops (standard ice pop molds hold 2 oz. or 4 T)

    2 c. unsweetened juice (any variety)

Pour juice into ice pop molds. Freeze.

Creamsicles

Yield: 8 pops

    1½ c. orange juice
    ½ c. vanilla ice cream, softened

Mix fruit juice with ice cream until thoroughly combined.
Pour mixture into ice pop molds. Freeze.

Homemade Granola Bars

Yield: 18 granola bars

3½ c. rolled oats
1 c. raisins or chopped dried fruit
1 c. finely chopped nuts
10 T. butter or margarine
¼ c. brown sugar
¼ c. honey
2 eggs, beaten
1 t. vanilla
½ t. cinnamon

Toast oats in a shallow pan at 350°F for 15 minutes.
Mix toasted oats with all remaining ingredients.
Press mixture into a well-greased 9- by 13-inch pan.
Bake at 350°F for 20 minutes.
Cool; cut into bars.

Create-a-Crunch

Select favorites from among the following ingredients. Using equal portions of each ingredient, toss to combine in a large bowl. Store in a covered container.

Popcorn	Cheerios	Soynuts
Peanuts	Kix	Pretzel Sticks
Unsalted Nuts	Mini-Wheats	Cheese crackers
Dried fruit, cut-up	Crispix	Sunflower seeds
Raisins	Corn Chex	Potato sticks

A small amount (¼ c.) of chocolate, butterscotch, or peanut butter morsels, or coconut could be added to your Create-a-Crunch mixture.

PUDDINGS AND GELATIN DESSERTS

Pudding Mix

Yield: 18–22 servings
      1 c. pudding mix = 4–5 servings

  3 c. nonfat dry milk powder
                or
  3 envelopes (1 quart) nonfat dry milk powder
¾ c. sugar
¾ c. cornstarch

Combine all ingredients and store in a tightly covered container.
To make pudding: Stir the dry mix thoroughly and measure 1 cup;
place in a small saucepan, gradually add 2 cups of water and the
flavor selected (see chart, Create-a-Pudding); and combine thoroughly. Cook over medium heat, stirring constantly until mixture
thickens and begins to boil. Pour into serving dishes and refrigerate.

Create-A-Pudding

Vanilla
1 c. pudding mix
2 c. water
1 t. vanilla
1 t. butter

Chocolate
 1 c. pudding mix
 2 c. water
½ t. vanilla
¼ c. chocolate chips (semisweet or milk chocolate)

Butterscotch
 1 c. pudding mix
 2 c. water
¼ c. butterscotch morsels

Peanut Butter
1 c. pudding mix
2 c. water
3 T. creamy peanut butter

Chocolate/Peanut Butter
1 c. pudding mix
2 c. water
2 T. creamy peanut butter
¼ c. chocolate chips (semisweet or milk chocolate)

Tapioca Pudding

Yield: 6 servings

3 T. quick-cooking tapioca
¼ c. sugar
1 egg, well beaten
2¾ c. milk
1 t. vanilla

Combine tapioca, sugar, egg, milk, and vanilla in a saucepan, and mix thoroughly to combine.
Let stand 5 minutes.
Cook over medium heat, stirring constantly, until mixture comes to a full boil.
Remove from heat; spoon into individual dishes or a covered bowl and let stand 20 minutes at room temperature.
Refrigerate until ready to use.

O.J. Tapioca

Yield: 6 servings

¼ c. quick-cooking tapioca
2½ c. orange juice
¼ c. sugar

Combine all ingredients and let stand 5 minutes.
Cook over medium heat, stirring constantly until mixture comes to a boil.

Remove from heat; spoon into dishes or bowl and let stand 20 minutes at room temperature.
Refrigerate until ready to use.

Apple-Graham Pudding

Yield: 6 servings

2 c. graham cracker crumbs
¼ c. granulated sugar
½ t. cinnamon
½ t. nutmeg
4 large apples, peeled, cored, and sliced
2 c. milk
2 eggs, slightly beaten

Combine crumbs, sugar, cinnamon, and nutmeg.
Place half the crumb mixture in the bottom of a 2-quart baking dish; cover with half the sliced apples.
Layer the rest of the crumbs over the apples and top crumbs with remaining apples.
Combine milk and eggs.
Slowly pour milk mixture over the apple and crumbs.
Bake at 400°F for 30 minutes.

Gel-O

Yield: 4 servings

1 envelope unflavored gelatin
½ c. cold water
2 T. sugar
1½ c. unsweetened fruit juice (any variety except pineapple)

Sprinkle gelatin over cold water in small saucepan; let stand 1–2 minutes; add sugar and fruit juice.
Cook over low heat, stirring constantly until gelatin dissolves (about 3 minutes).
Remove from heat, pour into serving dishes; chill until firm.

Gel-O plus Fruit

Yield: 6 servings

¾ c. fresh* or canned fruit
Gel-O

Prepare Gel-O recipe; chill until slightly thickened (about the consistency of unbeaten eggs); fold in fruit; spoon into serving dishes and chill until firm.

* Fresh pineapple cannot be used.

Appendices

Appendix I

Nutrients from A to Zinc

Calorie sources	Function	Food source
Carbohydrates	Supply energy and heat; help body to use protein and fat; many high-carbohydrate foods supply fiber too	Whole grain and enriched breads and cereals, fruit, honey, sugar, milk, dry peas and beans, potatoes, rice, pasta, noodles
Protein	Builds and maintains body tissues; supplies energy and heat	Meat, fish, poultry, milk, cheese, eggs, dried peas and beans, tofu, nuts, enriched and whole grain breads and cereals
Fat	Concentrated source of energy; saves protein for building tissues; carries fat-soluble vitamins; insulates body; protects organs	Butter, margarine, oils, salad dressing, mayonnaise, whole milk, cheese, ice cream, nuts, meat, poultry, fish, eggs, olives, avocado

Calorie sources	Function	Food source
Fat-Soluble Vitamins		
Vitamin A (retinol)	Promotes resistance to infection; needed for growth and maintenance of teeth, nails, hair, eyes, bones, and glands; helps eyes adjust from light to darkness	Liver, eggs, butter, margarine, milk, dark-green leafy and deep-yellow vegetables (spinach, broccoli, carrots, winter squash, sweet potatoes), apricots, mango
Vitamin D (ergosterol)	Helps absorption of the minerals, calcium and phosphorus and in their use in building bones and teeth	Vitamin D–fortified milk, margarine, fish liver oil, sunshine (ultraviolet rays) produce vitamin D in skin
Vitamin E	Aids the body's use of some vitamins and polyunsaturated fats; protects body substances	Salad oils (cottonseed, soy, corn, peanut, sunflower), margarine, whole grain breads and cereals, dark-green leafy vegetables, nuts, dried peas, and beans
Vitamin K	Helps blood clotting	Spinach, cabbage, cauliflower, liver
Water-Soluble Vitamins		
Vitamin C (ascorbic acid)	Helps hold body cells together; heals wounds; fights infection; used in tooth, bone, and blood formation	Citrus fruits (orange, grapefruit, tangerine, lemon, lime), cantaloupe, strawberries, tomato, papaya, cabbage, broccoli, green peppers, white and sweet potatoes

Calorie sources	Function	Food source
	Water-Soluble Vitamins	
Vitamin B_1 (thiamin)	Releases energy from food; needed for health of digestive and nervous system and maintenance of appetite	Whole grain and enriched breads and cereals, pork, liver, fish, poultry, dried peas and beans, potatoes
Vitamin B_2 (riboflavin)	Releases energy from food; needed for health of skin, tongue, lips, eyes, and nervous system	Milk, yogurt, cheese, liver, meat, fish, poultry, eggs, enriched and whole grain breads and cereals, deep-green leafy vegetables
Niacin	Helps body cells produce energy; maintains health of skin, tongue, digestive and nervous systems	Liver, peanuts, peanut butter, dried peas and beans, meat, poultry, fish, enriched and whole grain breads and cereals, potatoes, milk, yeast
Vitamin B_6 (pyridoxine)	Needed for body's use of carbohydrate, protein, and fat, for health of skin, lips, tongue, eyes, nerves, and circulatory system	Meat, poultry, fish, white and sweet potatoes, whole grain breads and cereals, milk, yeast
Vitamin B_{12} (cyancobalamin)	Needed for normal development of red blood cells; for health of digestive and nervous system	Meat, poultry, fish, liver, cheese, eggs, milk
Folic acid (folacin)	Needed for normal development of red blood cells; for normal use of proteins; development of genetic materials in body cells	Liver, dark-green leafy vegetables, meat, eggs, whole grain breads and cereals

Calorie sources	Function	Food source

Water-Soluble Vitamins

Calorie sources	Function	Food source
Pantothenic acid	Releases energy from carbohydrate; needed for normal use of fats and proteins; for health of nervous system	Eggs, whole grain breads and cereals, liver, peanuts, dry peas and beans, yeast
Biotin	Needed for use of carbohydrates, fats and proteins	Liver, meat, eggs, milk

Note: Choline, which transports fat in the body, is sometimes considered a vitamin. It can be made in the body from substances found in many foods. Inositol, another substance which has an uncertain function in the body, is sometimes grouped with the vitamins and is found in many foods.

Major Minerals

Calorie sources	Function	Food source
Calcium	Builds bones and teeth; helps blood clot; aids muscle and heart function and nerve response	Milk, yogurt, cheese, ice cream, deep-green leafy vegetables, canned salmon, and sardines eaten with bones, tofu
Phosphorus	Builds bones and teeth, aids in muscle function and nerve response; used in many reactions in body	Milk, cheese, meat, eggs, whole grain breads and cereals, nuts, dry peas and beans, soda, phosphate food additives
Magnesium	Builds bones and teeth; aids in nerve response and muscle function; used in many reactions in body	Whole grain breads and cereals, nuts, meat, milk, dry peas and beans

Calorie sources	Function	Food source
Major Minerals		
Sodium	Maintains normal body state; needed for nerves and muscle function	Table salt, milk, meat, eggs, baking powder, carrots, beets, celery, spinach, bouillon cubes
Potassium	Maintains normal body state; needed for nerve and muscle function	Fruits, vegetables, whole grain breads and cereals, dry peas and beans
Chlorine	Maintains normal body state; part of normal acid in stomach	Table salt
Sulfur	Helps rid body of toxins; part of body protein; used in many reactions in body	Meat, eggs, milk, cheese, nuts, dry peas and beans
Trace Minerals		
Iron	Builds red blood cells; helps release energy	Liver, meat, eggs, whole and enriched bread and cereals, dark-green leafy vegetables, nuts, dry peas and beans
Copper	Builds red blood cells; used to build bones and maintain nerves	Liver, meat, seafood, whole grain breads and cereals, dry peas and beans, nuts, cocoa
Iodine	Part of thyroid hormone	Seafood, iodized salt
Manganese	Needed for use of protein, sugar, and fats	Whole grain breads and cereals, soybeans, dry peas and beans, nuts, vegetables, fruits

Calorie sources	Function	Food source
	Trace Minerals	
Cobalt	Part of vitamin B_{12}; makes red blood cells	Meat, liver, milk, eggs, cheese
Zinc	Used in many cell activities; needed for wound healing and normal growth	Liver, meat, eggs, seafood, milk, whole grain breads and cereals
Molybdenum	Used in cell activities	Liver, milk, whole grain breads and cereals, leafy green vegetables, dry peas and beans
Fluoride	Builds strong teeth and bones	Tea, fluoridated water
Selenium	Helps to release energy, protects body substances	Seafood, meats, whole grain breads and cereal
Chromium	Helps body use carbohydrates	Meats, whole grain breads and cereals, yeast
Nickel	Used in cell activities	Whole grain breads and cereals, dry peas and beans, vegetables, fruits
Tin	Used in cell activities	Meats, whole grain breads and cereals, dry peas and beans, vegetables, fruits
Silicon	Forms bone and cartilage	Vegetables, fruit, whole grain cereals
Vanadium	Found in teeth	Whole grain cereal and breads, root vegetables, nuts, vegetable oils

Appendix II

NCHS Growth Charts

FOR BOYS AND GIRLS 2 TO 18 YEARS OF AGE

These charts to record the growth of the individual child were constructed by the National Center for Health Statistics in collaboration with the Centers for Disease Control. The charts are based on data from national probability samples representative of boys and girls in the general U.S. population. Their use will direct attention to unusual body size which may be due to disease or poor nutrition.

Take all measurements with the child in minimal indoor clothing and without shoes. Measure stature with the child standing. Use a scale to measure weight.

Then graph each measurement on the appropriate chart. Find the child's age on the horizontal scale; then follow a vertical line from that point to the horizontal level of the child's measurement (stature or weight). Where the two lines intersect, make a cross mark with a pencil. In graphing weight for stature, place the cross mark directly above the child's stature at the horizontal level of his weight.

Many factors influence growth. Therefore, growth data cannot be used alone to diagnose disease, but they do allow you to identify some unusual children.

Each chart contains a series of curved lines numbered to show selected percentiles. These refer to the rank of a measure in a group of 100. Thus, when a cross mark is on the 95th percentile line of weight for age it means that only five children among 100 of the corresponding age and sex have weight greater than that recorded.

BOYS FROM 2 TO 18 YEARS
WEIGHT FOR AGE

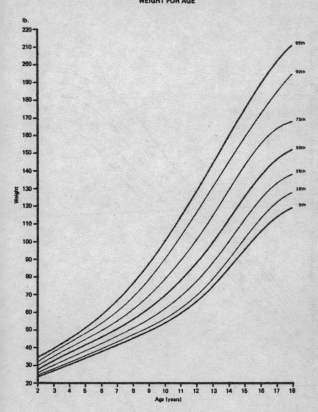

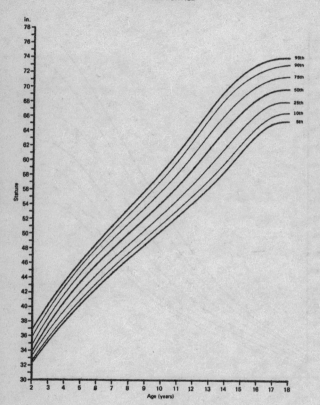

BOYS FROM 2 TO 18 YEARS

STATURE FOR AGE

(Courtesy of Mead Johnson Nutritional Division, Evansville, Indiana)

PRE-PUBERTAL BOYS FROM 2 TO 11½ YEARS

WEIGHT FOR STATURE

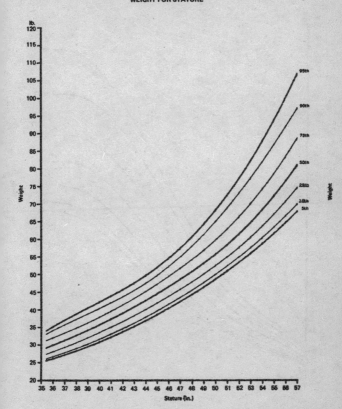

(Courtesy of Mead Johnson Nutritional Division, Evansville, Indiana)

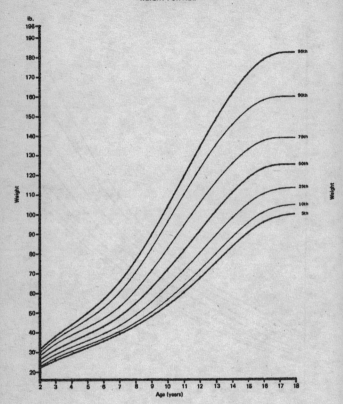

GIRLS FROM 2 TO 18 YEARS
WEIGHT FOR AGE

(Courtesy of Mead Johnson Nutritional Division, Evansville, Indiana)

GIRLS FROM 2 TO 18 YEARS
STATURE FOR AGE

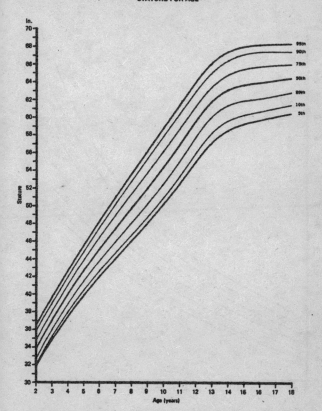

(Courtesy of Mead Johnson Nutritional Division, Evansville, Indiana)

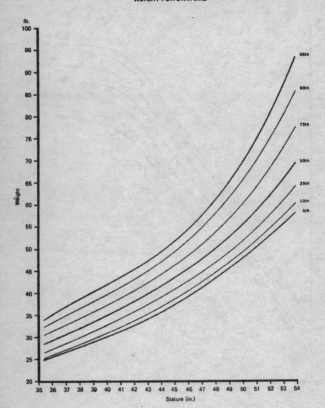

PRE-PUBERTAL GIRLS FROM 2 TO 10 YEARS

WEIGHT FOR STATURE

(Courtesy of Mead Johnson Nutritional Division, Evansville, Indiana)

Appendix III

Fast Foods

Note: Adapted from "Perspective on Fast Foods," *Dietetic Currents*, E. A. Young, Ross Laboratories, Columbus, Ohio, 1981; and *Food Values of Portions Commonly Used*, 13th ed. J. A. T. Pennington and H. N. Church, Harper & Row Publishers, 1980.

Nutritional Analyses of Fast Foods

(Dashes indicate no data available. X = Less than 2% US RDA; tr = trace.)

	Wt (g)	Energy (kcal)	PRO (g)	CHO (g)	Fat (g)	Chol (mg)	A (IU)	B1 (mg)	B2 (mg)	Nia. (mg)	B6 (mg)	B12 (µg)	C (mg)	D (IU)	Ca (mg)	Cu (mg)	Fe (mg)	K (mg)	Mg (mg)	P (mg)	Na (mg)	Zn (mg)	Moisture (g)	Crude Fiber (g)
ARBY'S®																								
Roast Beef	140	350	22	32	15	45	x	0.30	0.34	5	—	—	x	—	80	—	3.6	208	9	106	880	—	41	0.2
Beef and Cheese	168	450	27	36	28	55	x	0.38	0.43	6	—	—	x	—	200	—	4.5	210	9	202	1220	—	46	0.2
Super Roast Beef	263	620	30	61	28	85	x	0.42	0.43	7	—	—	x	—	100	—	4.0	360	15	355	1420	—	67	0.2
Junior Roast Beef	74	220	12	21	9	35	x	0.15	0.17	4	—	—	x	—	40	—	1.8	271	12	302	530	—	72	0.4
Ham & Cheese	154	380	23	33	17	60	x	0.75	0.34	5	—	—	x	—	200	—	5.4	578	25	377	1350	—	143	0.5
Turkey Deluxe	236	510	28	46	24	70	x	0.45	0.34	8	—	—	x	—	80	—	2.7	382	14	280	1220	—	80	0.3
Club Sandwich	252	560	30	43	30	100	x	0.68	0.43	7	—	—	x	—	200	—	3.6	612	26	445	1610	—	91	0.1

Source Consumer Affairs, Arby's, Inc. Atlanta, Georgia. Nutritional analysis by Technological Resources, Camden, New Jersey.

	Wt (g)	Energy (kcal)	PRO (g)	CHO (g)	Fat (g)	Chol (mg)	A (IU)	B1 (mg)	B2 (mg)	Nia. (mg)	B6 (mg)	B12 (µg)	C (mg)	D (IU)	Ca (mg)	Cu (mg)	Fe (mg)	K (mg)	Mg (mg)	P (mg)	Na (mg)	Zn (mg)	Moisture (g)	Crude Fiber (g)
BURGER CHEF®																								
Hamburger	91	244	11	29	9	27	114	0.17	0.16	2.7	0.16	0.26	1.2	—	45	0.08	2.0	183	26	106	—	1.6	70	0.8
Cheeseburger	104	290	14	29	13	39	267	0.18	0.21	2.7	0.21	0.36	1.2	—	132	0.10	3.2	386	53	202	—	5.6	209	1.3
Double Cheeseburger	145	420	24	30	22	77	431	0.23	0.22	4.8	0.31	0.73	1.2	—	243	0.04	3.2	397	49	355	—	1.2	195	1.8
Fish Filet	179	547	30	46	31	43	400	0.23	0.32	4.4	0.04	1.01	1.0	—	145	0.21	2.2	271	16	302	—	<0.1	29	0.6
Super Shef* Sandwich	252	563	29	44	30	105	754	0.31	0.40	6.0	0.45	0.87	9.3	—	205	0.21	4.5	578	40	377	—	<0.1	40	0.9
Big Shef* Sandwich	186	569	29	44	36	81	279	0.26	0.31	4.7	0.31	0.63	1.0	—	152	0.05	3.8	382	54	280	—	—	—	—
TOP Shef* Sandwich	138	661	41	54	38	134	273	0.35	0.47	8.1	0.56	1.16	1.0	—	194	0.13	5.4	612	50	445	—	—	—	—
Funmeal* Feast	316	545	15	55	30	27	123	0.25	0.21	4.6	0.16	0.26	12.8	—	61	0.24	2.8	688	—	183	—	—	—	—
Rancher* Platter*	316	640	32	53	42	106	1750*	0.29	0.38	8.6	0.61	1.01	23.5	—	66	0.38	5.3	1237	—	386	—	—	—	—
Mariner* Platter*	373	734	34	78	34	35	2069*	0.33	0.42	5.2	0.09	0.56	23.5	—	63	0.32	3.3	996	—	397	—	—	—	—
French Fries, small	68	250	3	28	13	0	0	0.07	0.04	1.7	—	—	11.5	—	9	0.16	0.9	473	—	62	—	—	—	—
French Fries, large	85	351	3	28	26	0	0	0.10	0.06	2.4	—	—	16.2	—	13	0.23	0.7	661	—	86	—	—	—	—
Vanilla Shake (12 oz)	336	380	13	60	10	40	387	0.16	0.66	0.5	0.1	1.77	—	—	497	—	0.3	622	40	392	—	1.3	—	—
Chocolate Shake (12 oz)	336	403	10	72	9	36	292	0.16	0.76	0.5	0.1	1.07	—	—	449	0.09	1.1	762	54	429	—	1.6	—	—
Hot Chocolate	—	198	8	23	8	30	288	0.93	0.39	0.3	0.1	0.79	2.1	—	271	—	0.7	436	50	245	—	1.1	—	—

*Includes salad.   Source Burger Chef Systems, Inc. Indianapolis, Indiana. Nutritional analysis from Handbook No. 8. Washington, US Dept of Agriculture.

	Wt (g)	Energy (kcal)	PRO (g)	CHO (g)	Fat (g)	Chol (mg)	A (IU)	B1 (mg)	B2 (mg)	Nia. (mg)	B6 (mg)	B12 (µg)	C (mg)	D (IU)	Ca (mg)	Cu (mg)	Fe (mg)	K (mg)	Mg (mg)	P (mg)	Na (mg)	Zn (mg)	Moisture (g)	Crude Fiber (g)
CHURCH'S FRIED CHICKEN®																								
White Chicken Portion	100	327	21	10	23	—	160	0.10	0.18	7.2	—	—	0.7	—	94	—	1.00	186	—	498	—	—	45	0.10
Dark Chicken Portion	100	305	22	7	21	—	140	0.10	0.27	5.3	—	—	1.0	—	15	—	1.3	206	—	475	—	—	48	0.20

Source: Church's Fried Chicken, San Antonio, Texas. Nutritional analysis by Medallion Laboratories, Minneapolis, Minnesota.

Nutritional Analyses of Fast Foods

(Dashes indicate no data available. X = Less than 2% US RDA; tr = trace.)

	WT (g)	Energy (kcal)	PRO (g)	CHO (g)	Fat (g)	Chol (mg)	A (IU)	B1 (mg)	B2 (mg)	Nia (mg)	B6 (mg)	B12 (µg)	C (mg)	D (IU)	Ca (mg)	Cu (mg)	Fe (mg)	K (mg)	Mg (mg)	P (mg)	Na (mg)	Zn (mg)	Moisture (g)	Crude Fiber (g)
DAIRY QUEEN®																								
Frozen Dessert	113	180	5	27	6	20	100	0.09	0.17	X	–	0.6	X	–	150	–	X	–	–	100	–	–	–	–
DO Cone, small	71	110	3	18	3	10	100	0.03	0.14	X	–	0.4	X	–	100	–	X	–	–	60	–	–	–	–
DO Cone, regular	142	230	6	35	7	20	300	0.09	0.26	X	–	0.8	X	–	200	–	X	–	–	150	–	–	–	–
DO Cone, large	213	340	9	52	10	30	400	0.15	0.39	X	–	1.2	X	–	200	–	X	–	–	200	–	–	–	–
DO Dip Cone, small	78	150	3	20	7	10	100	0.03	0.17	X	–	0.4	X	–	100	–	X	–	–	80	–	–	–	–
DO Dip Cone, regular	156	300	7	40	13	20	300	0.09	0.34	X	–	0.8	X	–	200	–	0.4	–	–	150	–	–	–	–
DO Dip Cone large	234	450	10	58	20	30	400	0.12	0.51	X	–	0.9	X	–	300	–	0.4	–	–	200	–	–	–	–
DO Sundae, small	106	170	4	30	4	15	100	0.03	0.17	X	–	0.5	X	–	100	–	0.7	–	–	100	–	–	–	–
DO Sundae, regular	177	290	6	51	7	20	300	0.06	0.26	X	–	0.8	X	–	200	–	1.1	–	–	150	–	–	–	–
DO Sundae, large	248	400	9	71	9	30	400	0.09	0.43	X	–	1.2	X	–	200	–	1.1	–	–	250	–	–	–	–
DO Malt, small	241	340	10	51	11	20	400	0.12	0.34	X	–	1.2	X	–	300	–	1.8	–	–	200	–	–	–	–
DO Malt, regular	418	600	15	89	20	50	750	0.12	0.60	0.8	–	1.8	2.4	60	500	–	1.8	–	–	400	–	–	–	–
DO Malt, large	588	840	22	125	28	70	750	0.12	0.85	1.2	–	2.4	3.6	140	600	–	5.4	–	–	600	–	–	–	–
DO Float	397	330	6	59	8	20	100	0.12	0.17	X	–	0.6	6	–	200	–	X	–	–	200	–	–	–	–
DO Banana Split	383	540	10	91	15	30	750	0.60	0.60	0.8	–	0.9	18	–	350	–	1.8	–	–	250	–	–	–	–
DO Parfait	284	460	10	81	15	30	400	0.43	0.43	0.4	–	1.2	X	–	300	–	1.8	–	–	250	–	–	–	–
DO Freeze	397	520	11	89	13	35	200	0.15	0.34	X	–	1.2	X	–	300	–	X	–	–	250	–	–	–	–
Mr. Misty* Freeze	411	500	9	85	12	30	200	0.12	0.17	X	–	0.6	X	–	300	–	X	–	–	200	–	–	–	–
"Dilly"* Bar	85	240	4	24	15	10	100	0.06	0.17	X	–	0.5	X	–	200	–	0.4	–	–	100	–	–	–	–
DQ Sandwich	60	140	3	24	4	10	–	0.03	0.14	X	–	0.2	X	–	60	–	0.4	–	–	60	–	–	–	–
Mr. Misty Kiss*	89	70	0	17	0	0	X	X	X	X	–	X	X	–	X	–	X	–	–	X	–	–	–	–
Brazier* Cheese Dog	113	330	15	24	19	–	–	0.15	0.18	3.3	0.07	1.22	11.0	23	168	0.08	1.6	–	24	182	939	1.9	–	–
Brazier* Chili Dog	128	330	13	25	20	–	–	0.15	0.23	3.0	0.17	1.29	11.0	23	158	0.13	1.8	–	38	133	868	1.8	–	–
Brazier* Dog	99	273	11	23	15	–	–	0.12	0.15	3.6	0.08	1.05	–	24	75	0.79	2.5	–	24	104	–	1.4	–	–
Fish Sandwich	177	400	20	41	17	–	100	0.15	0.26	3.0	0.16	1.50	–	40	60	0.08	1.1	–	24	250	–	0.3	–	–
Fish Sandwich w/Ch	177	440	24	39	21	–	tr	0.15	0.26	3.0	0.16	1.50	–	40	150	0.18	1.1	–	25	200	–	0.3	–	–
Super Brazier* Dog	182	518	20	41	30	–	tr	0.42	0.44	7.0	0.18	2.09	14.0	44	158	0.18	4.3	–	37	195	1552	2.8	–	–
Super Brazier* Dog w/Ch	203	593	26	43	36	–	tr	0.43	0.48	8.1	0.18	2.34	14.0	44	297	0.18	4.4	–	42	312	1986	3.5	–	–
Super Brazier* Chili Dog	210	555	23	42	33	–	tr	0.42	0.48	8.8	0.27	2.67	18.0	32	158	0.21	4.0	–	48	231	1640	2.8	–	–
Brazier* Fries, small	71	200	2	25	10	–	tr	0.06	0.16	0.8	0.16	–	3.6	–	tr	0.04	0.4	–	16	100	100	tr	–	–
Brazier* Fries, large	113	320	3	40	16	–	tr	0.09	0.30	1.2	0.30	–	4.8	–	tr	0.08	0.4	–	24	150	150	0.3	–	–
Brazier* Onion Rings	85	300	6	33	17	–	tr	0.09	0.08	0.8	0.08	–	2.4	–	20	0.04	0.4	–	16	60	60	0.3	–	–

Source: International Dairy Queen, Inc. Minneapolis, Minnesota. Nutritional analysis by Raltech Scientific Services, Inc. (formerly WARF), Madison Wisconsin (Nutritional analysis not applicable in the state of Texas)

Nutritional Analyses of Fast Foods

(Dashes indicate no data available. X = Less than 2% US RDA; tr = trace.)

	Wt (g)	Energy (kcal)	PRO (g)	CHO (g)	Fat (g)	Chel (mg)	A (IU)	B1 (mg)	B2 (mg)	Nia. (mg)	B6 (mg)	B12 (µg)	C (mg)	D (IU)	Ca (mg)	Cu (mg)	Fe (mg)	K (mg)	Mg (mg)	P (mg)	Na (mg)	Zn (mg)	Moisture (g)	Crude Fiber (g)
JACK IN THE BOX®																								
Hamburger	97	263	13	29	11	26	49	0.27	0.18	5.6	0.11	0.73	1.1	20	82	0.10	2.3	165	20	115	566	1.8	43	0.2
Cheeseburger	109	310	16	29	15	32	338	0.21	0.21	5.4	0.12	0.87	<1.7	20	172	0.10	2.6	177	22	194	877	2.3	47	0.2
Jumbo Jack™ Hamburger	246	551	28	45	29	53	246	0.47	0.32	11.6	0.30	2.68	<1.7	42	134	0.22	4.5	492	44	261	1134	4.2	139	0.7
Jumbo Jack™ Hamburger w/Ch	272	628	32	45	35	110	734	0.52	0.38	11.3	0.31	3.05	4.9	41	273	0.24	4.6	499	49	411	1666	4.8	153	0.8
Regular Taco	83	189	8	15	11	22	356	0.07	0.10	1.9	0.14	0.5	0.9	6	116	0.10	1.2	264	36	150	460	1.3	47	0.6
Super Taco	146	285	12	22	17	37	599	0.12	0.18	2.8	0.22	0.77	1.6	9	196	0.18	1.9	415	53	235	968	2.1	92	1.0
Moby Jack™ Sandwich	141	455	17	38	26	47	240	0.30	0.21	4.5	0.14	1.1	1.2	24	167	0.11	1.7	246	30	263	837	1.0	59	0.1
Breakfast Jack™ Sandwich	121	301	18	28	13	182	442	0.41	0.47	5.1	0.14	1.1	3.4	51	177	0.11	2.5	190	30	310	1037	1.8	59	0.1
French Fries	80	270	3	31	15	8	—	0.12	0.02	1.9	0.22	0.7	3.7	<1	19	0.07	0.7	423	27	88	128	0.4	29	0.6
Onion Rings	86	351	5	33	23	14	—	0.09	0.10	1.0	0.06	0.26	<1.2	<1	26	0.07	1.4	109	16	69	318	0.3	24	0.3
Apple Turnover	119	411	4	45	24	21	—	0.08	0.12	2.5	0.07	0.17	<1.2	<1	11	0.06	1.4	69	10	33	382	0.2	45	0.2
Vanilla Shake*	317	317	10	57	6	26	440	0.16	0.38	0.6	0.15	0.92	<3.2	43	349	0.13	0.6	599	38	312	229	1.0	243	0.3
Strawberry Shake*	326	323	11	55	7	14	426	0.16	0.46	0.6	0.20	1.25	<3.2	43	371	0.13	0.7	613	40	326	241	1.1	253	0.3
Chocolate Shake*	322	325	10	54	7	21	380	0.16	0.64	0.5	0.19	1.55	<3.5	44	348	0.13	0.7	676	53	328	270	1.1	247	0.3
Vanilla Shake	314	342	10	63	7	36	440	0.16	0.47	0.5	0.18	1.1	3.3	44	349	0.06	0.4	536	48	316	263	1.1	238	0.3
Strawberry Shake	328	380	11	63	10	33	426	0.16	0.60	0.6	0.18	0.92	3.3	44	351	0.07	0.4	556	47	316	268	1.2	242	0.3
Chocolate Shake	317	317	11	59	10	33	380	0.16	0.60	0.6	0.18	0.98	3.2	38	350	0.16	1.2	633	57	332	294	1.2	235	0.3
Ham & Cheese Omelette	174	425	21	32	23	355	766	0.45	0.70	3.0	0.18	1.44	1.7	64	260	0.14	4.0	237	29	397	975	2.3	94	0.2
Double Cheese Omelette	163	423	29	30	23	370	797	0.33	0.50	2.5	0.14	1.33	1.7	61	276	0.13	3.6	208	27	370	899	2.1	88	0.2
Ranchero Style Omelette	196	414	30	33	23	343	853	0.33	0.74	2.6	0.18	1.51	2.0	78	278	0.14	3.8	260	29	372	1098	2.0	117	0.4
French Toast	232	537	15	79	27	197	488	0.56	0.47	4.4	0.11	0.50	0.62	80	123	0.11	3.0	194	27	330	1130	1.9	78	0.9
Pancakes	232	626	16	79	27	85	488	0.63	0.62	4.5	0.22	0.56	<2.2	72	105	0.12	3.4	187	33	557	1670	1.9	104	0.7
Scrambled Eggs	267	719	26	55	44	259	694	0.69	0.56	5.2	0.34	1.31	<12.8	80	257	0.24	5.0	635	55	483	1110	3.0	137	1.3
KENTUCKY FRIED CHICKEN®																								
Original Recipe® Dinner*																								
Wing & Rib	322	603	30	48	32	133	25.5	0.22	0.19	10.0	—	—	36.6	—	—	—	—	—	—	—	—	—	—	—
Wing & Thigh	341	661	35	38	48	172	25.5	0.24	0.27	8.4	—	—	36.6	—	—	—	—	—	—	—	—	—	—	—
Drum & Thigh	346	643	35	46	35	180	25.5	0.25	0.32	8.5	—	—	36.6	—	—	—	—	—	—	—	—	—	—	—
Extra Crispy Dinner*																								
Wing & Rib	349	755	33	60	43	132	25.5	0.31	0.29	10.4	—	—	36.6	—	—	—	—	—	—	—	—	—	—	—
Wing & Thigh	371	812	33	58	48	176	25.5	0.31	0.35	10.3	—	—	36.6	—	—	—	—	—	—	—	—	—	—	—
Drum & Thigh	376	765	38	55	46	183	25.5	0.32	0.38	10.4	—	—	36.6	—	—	—	—	—	—	—	—	—	—	—
Mashed Potatoes	85	64	2	12	1	<18	<18	0.01	0.02	0.8	—	—	4.9	—	—	—	—	—	—	—	—	—	—	—
Gravy	14	—	<1	1	1	<3	<3	<0.01	0.01	0.1	—	—	<0.2	—	—	—	—	—	—	—	—	—	—	—
Cole Slaw	91	122	1	13	8	7	<5	0.04	0.04	1.0	—	—	0.3	—	—	—	—	—	—	—	—	—	—	—
Rolls	21	61	2	11	1	7	<3	0.10	0.07	—	—	—	0.3	—	—	—	—	—	—	—	—	—	—	—
Corn (5.5-inch ear)	135	169	5	31	3	X	162	0.12	—	1.2	—	—	2.6	—	—	—	—	—	—	—	—	—	—	—

*Special formula for shakes sold in California, Arizona, Texas and Washington. Source: Jack-in-the-Box. Nutritional analysis by Raltech Scientific Services, Inc. (formerly WARF), Madison, Wisconsin.

*Includes two pieces of chicken, mashed potato and gravy, cole slaw, and roll. Source: Kentucky Fried Chicken, Inc. Louisville, Kentucky. Nutritional analysis by Raltech Scientific Services, Inc. (formerly WARF), Madison, Wisconsin.

Nutritional Analyses of Fast Foods

(Dashes indicate no data available. X = Less than 2% US RDA; tr=trace.)

Food	Wet (g)	Energy (kcal)	PRO (g)	CHO (g)	Fat (g)	Chol (mg)	A (IU)	B1 (mg)	B2 (mg)	Nia (mg)	B6 (mg)	B12 (µg)	C (mg)	D (IU)	Ca (mg)	Cu (mg)	Fe (mg)	K (mg)	Mg (mg)	P (mg)	Na (mg)	Zn (mg)	Moisture (g)	Crude Fiber (g)
LONG JOHN SILVER'S®																								
Fish w/Batter (3 pc)	136	366	22	21	22	—	97	0.47	0.44	3.8	—	—	—	—	—	—	—	—	—	—	—	—	—	—
Fish w/Batter (2 pc)	207	549	30	32	32	—	164	0.28	0.49	2.6	—	—	—	—	—	—	—	—	—	—	—	—	—	—
Treasure Chest*	143	506	30	32	32	—	257	0.26	0.36	2.3	—	—	—	—	—	—	—	—	—	—	—	—	—	—
Chicken Planks* (4 pc)	166	457	27	35	23	—	<32	0.27	0.11	2.1	—	—	—	—	—	—	—	—	—	—	—	—	—	—
Peg Legs* w/Batter (5 pc)	125	350	22	26	23	—	<14	0.08	0.47	0.8	—	—	—	—	—	—	—	—	—	—	—	—	—	—
Ocean Scallops (6 pc)	120	283	11	30	13	—	530	0.39	0.37	6.5	—	—	—	—	—	—	—	—	—	—	—	—	—	—
Shrimp w/Batter (6 pc)	88	268	8	30	13	—	345	0.25	0.15	3.8	—	—	—	—	—	—	—	—	—	—	—	—	—	—
Breaded Oysters (6 pc)	156	441	13	53	19	—	82	0.25	0.18	4.0	—	—	—	—	—	—	—	—	—	—	—	—	—	—
Breaded Clams (6 pc)	142	617	18	61	34	—	133	0.32	0.28	6.5	—	—	—	—	—	—	—	—	—	—	—	—	—	—
Fish Sandwich	193	337	22	49	31	—	660	0.26	0.28	7.4	—	—	—	—	—	—	—	—	—	—	—	—	—	—
French Fries	85	288	4	33	16	—	<17	0.12	0.02	2.3	—	—	—	—	—	—	—	—	—	—	—	—	—	—
Cole Slaw	113	138	1	16	8	—	<34	0.02	0.02	0.2	—	—	—	—	—	—	—	—	—	—	—	—	—	—
Corn on the Cob (1 ear)	150	176	5	29	4	—	114	0.03	0.02	0.4	—	—	—	—	—	—	—	—	—	—	—	—	—	—
Hushpuppies (3)	45	153	3	20	7	—	<27	0.03	0.02	0.2	—	—	—	—	—	—	—	—	—	—	—	—	—	—
Clam Chowder (8 oz)	170	107	5	15	3	—	42	0.26	0.09	2.9	—	—	—	—	—	—	—	—	—	—	—	—	—	—

Source: Long John Silver's Food Shoppes, Lexington, Kentucky. Nutritional analysis by L. V. Packett, PhD. The Department of Nutrition and Food Science, University of Kentucky.

Food	Wet (g)	Energy (kcal)	PRO (g)	CHO (g)	Fat (g)	Chol (mg)	A (IU)	B1 (mg)	B2 (mg)	Nia (mg)	B6 (mg)	B12 (µg)	C (mg)	D (IU)	Ca (mg)	Cu (mg)	Fe (mg)	K (mg)	Mg (mg)	P (mg)	Na (mg)	Zn (mg)	Moisture (g)	Crude Fiber (g)
McDONALD'S®																								
Egg McMuffin®	138	327	19	31	15	229	530	0.39	0.44	3.8	0.21	0.75	<1.4	46	226	0.12	4.0	168	26	322	885	1.9	70.7	0.1
English Muffin, Buttered	63	186	5	30	5	13	160	0.28	0.03	2.6	0.04	0.02	4.7	14	117	0.09	1.5	71	13	105	318	0.5	21.7	0.1
Hotcakes w/Butter & Syrup	214	500	8	94	10	47	257	0.26	0.36	2.3	0.12	0.19	0.5	31	103	0.11	2.3	187	28	249	1070	0.5	97.8	0.2
Sausage (Pork)	53	206	9	tr	19	43	<32	0.27	0.11	2.1	0.18	0.53	1.7	65	16	0.05	0.8	127	13	67	615	1.7	22.9	0.2
Scrambled Eggs	98	180	13	3	13	349	652	0.08	0.47	0.8	0.13	0.93	<0.1	65	65	0.06	2.4	247	13	264	205	1.3	68.1	<0.1
Hashbrown Potatoes	55	125	2	14	7	7	<14	0.06	<0.01	0.8	0.13	0.01	1.1	5	5	0.04	0.6	247	13	67	325	0.3	30.9	0.3
Big Mac®	204	563	26	41	33	86	349	0.39	0.37	6.5	0.27	1.8	2.2	33	157	0.11	4.0	237	38	314	1010	4.7	100.4	0.6
Cheeseburger	115	307	15	30	14	37	377	0.25	0.18	3.8	0.12	0.91	1.6	13	132	0.10	2.3	156	19	205	767	2.6	108.4	0.2
Hamburger	102	255	12	30	10	37	349	0.25	0.18	4.0	0.12	0.81	1.7	13	51	0.11	2.3	142	19	120	520	2.1	48.0	0.3
Quarter Pounder®	166	424	24	33	22	67	231	0.32	0.28	6.5	0.27	0.88	1.7	25	98	0.17	4.1	322	37	249	735	5.7	83.7	0.3
Quarter Pounder® w/Ch	194	524	30	33	31	96	349	0.32	0.28	7.4	0.27	2.15	2.7	25	219	0.17	4.3	341	41	382	1236	5.7	96.0	0.7
Filet-O-Fish®	139	432	14	37	25	47	230	0.26	0.10	2.6	0.10	0.82	1.4	10	93	0.13	1.7	150	27	229	781	0.5	59.5	0.1
Regular Fries	68	220	3	26	9	9	<17	0.12	0.02	2.3	0.23	<0.03	12.5	2	14	0.03	0.6	564	27	74	109	0.3	25.4	0.5
Apple Pie	85	253	2	29	14	12	<34	0.02	0.02	0.2	0.02	<0.04	<0.8	14	14	0.06	0.6	39	6	27	398	0.2	38.9	0.3
Cherry Pie	88	260	2	32	14	13	114	0.03	0.02	0.4	0.02	<0.02	<0.8	10	16	0.05	1.2	39	7	27	427	0.2	38.9	<0.3
McDonaldland® Cookies	67	308	4	49	11	10	<27	0.23	0.04	2.9	0.29	0.03	2.9	10	12	0.03	0.8	52	11	74	358	0.3	2.2	0.1
Chocolate Shake	291	383	10	66	9	30	349	0.12	0.44	0.5	0.13	1.16	2.9	44	320	0.19	0.8	580	49	335	300	1.4	203.0	0.3
Strawberry Shake	290	362	9	62	9	32	377	0.12	0.70	0.4	0.14	1.16	4.1	377	322	0.07	0.2	423	31	313	207	1.2	207.1	<0.3
Vanilla Shake	291	352	9	60	8	31	349	0.12	0.31	0.4	0.13	1.19	3.2	26	329	0.12	0.2	410	35	307	201	1.0	211.3	<0.3
Hot Fudge Sundae	164	310	7	46	11	18	230	0.07	0.31	1.1	0.13	0.7	2.5	35	215	0.09	0.4	338	30	236	175	0.9	97.9	0.2
Caramel Sundae	165	328	7	53	10	25	279	0.07	0.35	1.0	0.13	0.7	3.6	16	200	0.13	0.4	290	30	230	195	0.9	93.2	0.2
Strawberry Sundae	164	289	7	46	9	20	230	0.07	0.30	1.0	0.05	0.6	2.8	16	174	0.11	0.4	290	28	80	96	0.8	101.0	0.2

Source: McDonald's Corporation, Oak Brook, Illinois. Nutritional analysis by Raltech Scientific Services, Inc. (formerly WARF), Madison, Wisconsin

Nutritional Analyses of Fast Foods

(Dashes indicate no data available. X = less than 2% US RDA; tr = trace.)

	Wt (g)	Energy (kcal)	PRO (g)	CHO (g)	Fat (g)	Chol (mg)	A (IU)	B1 (mg)	B2 (mg)	Nia. (mg)	B6 (mg)	B12 (µg)	C (mg)	D (IU)	Ca (mg)	Cu (mg)	Fe (mg)	K (mg)	Mg (mg)	P (mg)	Na (mg)	Zn (mg)	Caf-feine (mg)	Sac-char (mg)
TACO BELL®																								
Bean Burrito	166	343	11	48	12	—	1657	0.37	0.22	2.2	—	—	15.2	—	98	—	2.8	235	—	173	272	—	—	—
Beef Burrito	184	466	30	37	21	—	1675	0.30	0.39	7.0	—	—	15.2	—	83	—	4.6	320	—	288	300	—	—	—
Beefy Tostada	184	291	19	21	15	—	3450	0.16	0.27	3.3	—	—	12.7	—	208	—	3.4	277	—	265	138	—	—	—
Bellbeefer™	123	221	15	23	7	—	2961	0.15	0.20	3.7	—	—	10.0	—	40	—	2.6	183	—	140	231	—	—	—
Bellbeefer™ w/Ch	137	278	19	23	12	—	3146	0.16	0.27	3.7	—	—	10.0	—	147	—	2.7	195	—	208	330	—	—	—
Burrito Supreme™	225	457	21	43	22	—	3462	0.33	0.35	4.7	—	—	16.0	—	121	—	3.8	350	—	245	367	—	—	—
Combination Burrito	175	404	21	43	16	—	1666	0.34	0.31	4.6	—	—	15.2	—	91	—	3.7	278	—	230	300	—	—	—
Enchirito™	207	454	25	42	21	—	1178	0.31	0.37	4.7	—	—	9.5	—	259	—	3.8	491	—	338	1175	—	—	—
Pintos 'N Cheese	158	168	11	21	5	—	3123	0.26	0.16	0.9	—	—	9.3	—	150	—	2.3	307	—	210	102	—	—	—
Taco	83	186	15	14	8	—	120	0.09	0.16	2.9	—	—	0.2	—	120	—	2.5	143	—	175	79	—	—	—
Tostada	138	179	9	25	6	—	3152	0.18	0.15	0.8	—	—	9.7	—	191	—	2.3	186	—	186	101	—	—	—

Sources: 1) Menu Item Portions, Taco Bell Co. July 1976 2) Adams CF Nutritive value of American foods in common units, in *Handbook No. 456*, Washington USDA Agricultural Research Service. November 1975 3) Church EF, Church HN (eds) *Food Values of Portions Commonly Used*, ed 12 Philadelphia JB Lippincott Co. 1975 4) Valley Baptist Medical Center. Food Service Department *Descriptions of Mexican-American Foods* Fort Atkinson, Wisconsin NASCO

	Wt (g)	Energy (kcal)	PRO (g)	CHO (g)	Fat (g)	Chol (mg)	A (IU)	B1 (mg)	B2 (mg)	Nia. (mg)	B6 (mg)	B12 (µg)	C (mg)	D (IU)	Ca (mg)	Cu (mg)	Fe (mg)	K (mg)	Mg (mg)	P (mg)	Na (mg)	Zn (mg)	Caf-feine (mg)	Sac-char (mg)
WENDY'S®																								
Single Hamburger	200	470	26	34	26	70	94	0.24	0.36	5.8	—	—	0.6	—	84	—	5.3	—	—	239	774	4.8	110.6	0.8
Double Hamburger	285	670	44	34	40	125	128	0.43	0.54	10.6	—	—	1.5	—	138	—	8.2	—	—	364	980	8.4	162.1	1.1
Triple Hamburger	360	850	65	33	51	265	128	0.47	0.68	14.7	—	—	2.0	—	104	—	10.7	—	—	525	1217	13.5	204.6	1.0
Single w/Cheese	240	580	33	41	34	90	221	0.38	0.43	6.3	—	—	0.7	—	228	—	5.4	—	—	315	1085	5.5	133.4	1.3
Double w/Cheese	325	800	50	41	48	155	472	0.75	0.84	11.4	—	—	2.3	—	177	—	10.2	—	—	489	1414	10.1	179.2	1.3
Triple w/Cheese	400	1040	72	35	68	225	—	0.80	1.20	15.1	—	—	3.4	—	371	—	10.9	—	—	712	1848	14.3	216.4	1.6
Chili	250	230	19	21	9	25	1188	0.14	0.07	3.4	—	—	6.4	—	83	—	4.4	—	—	168	1065	3.7	195.9	2.3
French Fries	120	330	5	41	16	5	40	0.20	0.25	X	—	—	—	—	16	—	1.2	—	—	196	112	0.5	54.9	1.2
Frosty	250	390	9	54	16	45	355	0.60	0.60	X	0	X	0.7	—	270	—	0.9	—	—	278	247	1.0	169.8	0.0

Source: Wendy's International, Inc. Dublin, Ohio Nutritional analysis by Medallion Laboratories, Minneapolis, Minnesota.

	Wt (g)	Energy (kcal)	PRO (g)	CHO (g)	Fat (g)	Chol (mg)	A (IU)	B1 (mg)	B2 (mg)	Nia. (mg)	B6 (mg)	B12 (µg)	C (mg)	D (IU)	Ca (mg)	Cu (mg)	Fe (mg)	K (mg)	Mg (mg)	P (mg)	Na (mg)	Zn (mg)	Caf-feine (mg)	Sac-char (mg)
PIZZA																								
Pizza, cheese 1 slice	100	239	13	28	8	—	141	0.16	0.24	1.7	—	—	—	—	225	—	1.3	233	33	215	585	—	—	—
Pizza, thick crust, 10 inch	417	919	46	156	12	—	—	—	—	—	—	—	—	—	579	—	5.2	947	156	637	2265	—	—	—
Cheese pizza, thin crust 10 inch	336	718	37	98	19	—	—	—	—	—	—	—	—	—	710	—	2.2	570	79	669	2232	—	—	—
Pepperoni pizza 1 slice	100	234	8	29	9	—	560	0.09	0.12	1.5	—	—	9	—	17	—	1.2	168	—	92	729	—	—	—

Nutritional Analyses of Fast Foods

(Dashes indicate no data available. X = Less than 2% US RDA; tr = trace.)

							VITAMINS								MINERALS									
BEVERAGES	Wt (g)	Energy (kcal)	PRO (g)	CHO (g)	Fat (g)	Chol (mg)	A (IU)	B1 (mg)	B2 (mg)	Nia. (mg)	B6 (mg)	B12 (µg)	C (mg)	D (IU)	Ca (mg)	Cu (mg)	Fe (mg)	K (mg)	Mg (mg)	P (mg)	Na (mg)	Zn (mg)	Caffeine (mg)	Sac-char. (mg)
Coffee*	180	2	tr	tr	tr	tr	0	0	tr	0.5	-	-	0	-	4	-	-	65	-	7	2	-	100†	0
Tea*	180	2	tr	1	tr	-	0	0	0.04	0.1	-	-	1	-	5	-	-	-	-	4	-	-	40†	0
Orange Juice	183	82	1	20	tr	-	366	0.17	0.02	0.6	-	-	82.4	-	17	-	0.2	340	-	29	2	-	0	0
Chocolate Milk	250	213	9	28	9	-	330	0.08	0.40	0.3	-	-	3.0	-	278	-	0.2	365	18	235	118	-	-	0
Skim Milk	245	88	9	13	tr	-	10	0.09	0.44	0.2	-	-	2.0	-	296	-	0.5	355	-	233	127	-	-	0
Whole Milk	244	159	9	12	9	27	342	0.07	0.41	0.2	-	-	2.4	100	288	-	tr	351	32	227	122	-	-	0
Coca-Cola*	246	96	0	24	0	0	-	-	-	-	-	-	-	-	-	-	-	-	-	40	20‡	-	28	0
Fanta* Ginger Ale	244	84	0	21	0	0	-	-	-	-	-	-	-	-	-	-	-	-	-	-	30‡	-	0	0
Fanta* Grape	247	114	0	29	0	0	-	-	-	-	-	-	-	-	-	-	-	-	-	-	21‡	-	0	0
Fanta* Orange	248	117	0	30	0	0	-	-	-	-	-	-	-	-	-	-	-	-	-	-	21‡	-	0	0
Fanta* Root Beer	246	103	0	27	0	0	-	-	-	-	-	-	-	-	-	-	-	-	-	-	23‡	-	0	0
Mr. Pibb*	245	95	0	25	0	0	-	-	-	-	-	-	-	-	-	-	-	-	-	29	23‡	-	27	0
Mr. Pibb* w/o Sugar	245	1	0	tr	0	0	-	-	-	-	-	-	-	-	-	-	-	-	-	28	37‡	-	38	76
Sprite*	245	95	0	24	0	0	-	-	-	-	-	-	-	-	-	-	-	-	-	-	42‡	-	0	0
Sprite* w/o Sugar	236	3	0	0	0	0	-	-	-	-	-	-	-	-	-	-	-	-	-	-	42‡	-	0	57
Tab*	236	0	0	0	0	0	-	-	-	-	-	-	-	-	-	-	-	-	-	30	30‡	-	30	74
Fresca*	236	2	0	0	0	0	-	-	-	-	-	-	-	-	-	-	-	-	-	-	38	-	0	54

*6-oz serving: all other data are for 8-oz serving. †Caffeine content depends on strength of beverage. ‡Value when bottling water with average sodium content (12 mg/6 oz) is used. Sources: 1) Adams CF: Nutritive value of American foods in common units, in Handbook No. 456. Washington, USDA Agricultural Research Service, November 1975; 2) The Coca-Cola Company, Atlanta, Georgia, January 1977; 3) American Hospital Formulary Service, Washington, American Society of Hospital Pharmacists, Section 28:20, March 1978.

Bibliography

Alfano, M. C., Ed., *Changing Perspectives in Nutrition and Caries Research*. American Academy of Pedodontics, N.Y.: Medcom, Inc., 1979.

Barhart, W. E. et al., Dentifrice usage and ingestion among four age groups. *Journal of Dental Research* 53:1317, 1974.

Bo-Linn, G. W. et al., Purging and calorie absorption in bulimic patients and normal women. *Annals of Internal Medicine* 99:14, 1983.

Brace, E. R., *The Pediatric Guide to Drugs and Vitamins*. New York: Dell, 1982.

Bradley, R. L., Effect of light on alteration of nutritional value and flavor of milk: A review. *Journal of Food Protection* 43:314, April 1980.

Buskirke, Elsworth, Diet and athletic performance. *Postgraduate Medicine* 61(1):229, 1977.

Caffeine, The Institute of Nutrition of the University of North Carolina, 311 Pittsboro Street, 256-H, Chapel Hill, North Carolina 27514, 1981.

Christophersen, E. R. and Hall, C. L., Eating patterns and associated problems encountered in normal children. *Comprehensive Pediatric Nursing* 3(1):1, October 1978.

Cohen, S. A. et al., Chronic nonspecific diarrhea. *American Journal of Diseases of the Child* 133:490, May 1979.

Consumption of Salted Snack Foods by U.S. Teenagers, Michigan State University. *Agricultural Experiment Station Report* 439: Home and Family Living, March 1982.

Cook, J. D., Nutritional anemia. *Contemporary Nutrition* 8(4), 1983.

Costill, David L., Sports Nutrition: The role of carbohydrates. *Nutrition News* 41(1), February 1978.

Crosby, W. H., Prescribing iron? Think safety. *Archives of Internal Medicine* 138:766, May 1978.

Curatolo, P. W. and Robertson, D., The health consequences of caffeine. *Annals of Internal Medicine* 98(part 1):641, May 1983.

Diarrhea from herbal teas. *Pediatric Alert* August 3, 1978, p. 70.

Edible T.V.: Your Child and Food Commercials. U.S. Government Printing Office, 1977.

Faulty eating habits: Effect on children. *Nutrition and the M.D.* 5(8):1, August 1979.

Fogoros, R. N., Runners trots: Gastrointestinal disturbances in runners. *Journal of the American Medical Association* 243:1743, 1980.

For the Preschooler, Volumes I, II, III. Washington State Department of Social and Health Services, 1981.

Gallo, A. E. and Connor, J. M., Advertising and American food consumption patterns. *National Food Review* summer 1982, p. 2.

Giannini, A. J. and Slaby, A. E., Ascorbic acid: A speculation on oranges, puberty, marriage contracts and frozen foods. *M.D.*, May 1981, p. 51.

Guinta, G. L., Dental erosion from chewable vitamin C. *Journal of the American Dental Association* 107:253, 1983.

Hannigan, K. J., Aseptic package report: The consumer likes it! *Food Engineering* 54:53, February 1982.

Hagerman, Gene R., Nutrition in part-time athletes. *Nutrition and the M.D.* VII(8):August 1, 1981.

Hockman, H., Is eating hazardous to your skin? *Environmental Nutrition* 3(4), 1980.

Hudnall, Marsha, Hypoglycemia: Myths and realities. *American Council on Science and Health* 2(5):4, 1981.

Iron Deficiency in Infancy and Childhood. The Nutrition Foundation, 888 17th St. N.W., Washington, D.C. 20006.

Juvenile hypertension. *M.D.* 23(2):53, 1979.

Leibel, R. L. Behavior and biochemical correlates of iron deficiency: A review. *Journal of the American Dietetic Association* 71:399, 1977.

Ling, L. and McCamman, S. P., Dietary treatment of diarrhea and constipation in infants and children. *Comprehensive Pediatric Nursing* 3(4):17, October 1978.

Lipton, M. A. and Mayo, J. P., Diet and hyperkinesis: An update. *Journal of the American Dietetic Association* 83(2):132, August 1983.

Longseth, Lillian, Soft drinks: The great American beverage. *ACSH News and Views* May/June 1982, p. 10.

Manual of Pediatric Nutrition: Twin Cities District Dietetic Association, Minneapolis, 1983.

Monopoly on the cereal shelves? *Consumer Reports* 46(2):76, February 1981.

Morgan, K. J., The role of snacking in the American diet. *Contemporary Nutrition* 7(9), September 1982.

Morgan, K. J. et al., The role of breakfast in nutrient intake of 5- to 12-year-old children. *American Journal of Clinical Nutrition* 34:1418, July 1981.

Moskowitz, H. R., Searching for good taste in food. *Professional Nutritionist* 12(4):7, Fall 1980.

Nelson, Ralph A., What should athletes eat? Unmixing folly and facts. *The Physician and Sports Medicine* November 1975, p. 67.

Nutrition for Athletes—A Handbook for Coaches. American Alliance for Health, Physical Education, and Recreation, 1210 Sixteenth St. N.W., Washington, D.C. 20036.

Nutritional Concerns during Adolescence. *Dairy Council Digest* 52(2):1, 1981.

Pao, E. M., *Eating Patterns and Food Frequencies of Children in the United States.* Consumer Nutrition Center, Human Nutrition Science and Education Administration, U.S. Department of Agriculture, Hyattsville, Maryland 20782, October 1980.

Pochi, P. E., Hormones, retinoids and acne. *New England Journal of Medicine* 308(17):1024, 1983.

Pollitt, E. et al., Brief fasting, stress, and cognition in children. *The American Journal of Clinical Nutrition* 34:1526, August 1981.

Pollitt, E. and Leibel, R. L., Iron deficiency and behavior. *Journal of Pediatrics* 88:372, 1976.

Randolph, P. M., The role of diet and nutrition in dental health and disease. *Nutrition News* 44(1):1, February 1981.

Rapp, C. E., The adolescent patient. *Annals of Internal Medicine* 99:52, 1983.

Ravry, M. J. R., Dietetic food diarrhea. *Journal of the American Medical Association* 244(3):270, 1980.

Read, M. S., Malnutrition, hunger, and behavior. *Journal of the American Dietetic Association* 63:386, October 1973.

Schachtele, C. F., Bacteria, diet, and the prevention of dental caries, Part I. *Contemporary Nutrition* 5(7), July 1980.

Schachtele, C. F., Bacteria, diet, and the prevention of dental caries, Part II. *Contemporary Nutrition* 5(8), August 1980.

Schwabe, A. D. et al., Anorexia nervosa. *Annals of Internal Medicine* 94:371, 1981.

Storz, N. S., Body weight concepts of adolescent girls in the home economics classroom. *Journal of Home Economics* 74(1):41, 1982.

Streeter, S. K. et al., Television and human values: A case for cooperation. *Journal of Home Economics* Summer 1982, p. 18.

The Gallup Study of Vitamin Use in the United States, Survey VI, Volume I. The Gallup Organization, Princeton, New Jersey, 1982.

Timbie, D. J., Sechrist, L., and Keeney, P. G., Application of high pressure liquid chromatography to the study of variables affecting theobromine and caffeine concentrations in cocoa beans. *Journal of Food Science* 43, 1978.

Torre, C. T., Nutritional needs of adolescents. *The American Journal of Maternal/Child Nursing* March/April 1977, p. 118.

Travis, Susan, Food, nutrition and teenagers. *Professional Perspectives* July 1982.

Viewpoint, Soda manufacturers wage war. *Environmental Nutrition Newsletter* 6(8):5, August 1983.

Vitorisek, Sharon H., Is More Better? *Nutrition Today* 14(6):10, 1979.

Way, W. L., Food-related behavior on prime-time television. *Journal of Nutrition Education* 15(3):105, 1983.

Wei, S. H. Y., Nutrition, diet, fluoride and dental health. *Pediatric Basics* 30:4, 1981.

Which Cereal for Breakfast? *Consumer Reports* 46(2):68, February 1981.

Whitney, E. N., and Hamilton, E. M. N., *Understanding Nutrition*. St. Paul: West Publishing Co., 1981.

Yogman, M. W., and Zeisel, S. H., Diet and sleep patterns and newborn infants. *New England Journal of Medicine* 309(19):1147, 1983.

You Should Know . . . about Sweeteners. Cornell Cooperative Extension, Cornell University, October 1982.

Index

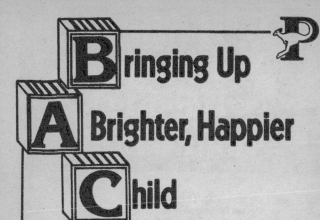

Helping Your Children With Divorce

by Dr. Edward Teyber

With an Introduction by Dr. Leo F. Buscaglia

A compassionate guide for parents raising children in the aftermath of divorce. Dr. Edward Teyber, a family therapist, uses case studies and family scenarios to illustrate his unique techniques for resolving divorce conflicts. He also provides practical, supportive advice on the best way to identify or deal with:

- **Your children's abandonment fears**
- **Children who choose sides between parents**
- **The absentee father**
- **Burdening your children with your emotional needs**
- **Predictable discipline problems**
- *And many other critical issues*